HABITS NOT DIETS

The Secret to Lifetime Weight Control

James M. Ferguson, M.D.

BULL PUBLISHING COMPANY
Palo Alto, California 94302

Bull Publishing Company
P.O. Box 208
Palo Alto, California 94302-0208
(415) 322-2855

ISBN 0-915950-85-5

Printed in the United States

Distributed to the trade by:
Publishers Group West
4065 Hollis Street
Emeryville, California 94608

Library of Congress Cataloging-in-Publication Data

Ferguson, James Mecham, 1941–
Habits, not diets.

Bibliography: p.
Includes index.
1. Reducing—Psychological aspects. 2. Behavior therapy. 3. Food habits. I. Title.
RM222.2.F4267 1988 613.2′5 88-7378
ISBN 0-915950-85-5

Design by: Robb Pawlak
Production Manager: Helen O'Donnell

CONTENTS

CONTENTS

FROM THE PREFACE TO THE FIRST EDITION

The last ten years have witnessed a marked change in our views about the eating which leads to obesity. The origins of such eating had long been assumed to lie in some defective inner state, metabolic or psychological, and the control of obesity lay in the remedying of that defect. The result was a vast outpouring of appetite-suppressant medication and a no less intense program of exhorting obese people to exercise will power and self-denial.

Two developments shifted our attention from defects within the person to the social environment around him. One was understanding the powerful influence of social factors on obesity. The other was the introduction of behavior modification.

The application of behavior modification to the treatment of obesity was a natural. For it is ideally suited to analyzing just how social factors exert their influence, and it has proceeded to do just that. Only eight years after its introduction, a short time in the history of psychotherapy research, behavior modification has sparked a veritable explosion of research on the treatment of obesity. Within the past four years alone, over 30 reports have been devoted to applications of behavior modification in this area. They have established beyond a doubt these techniques are more effective than traditional weight reduction measures; and they are elucidating just which of the many behavioral techniques are the most effective.

The explosion of research on behavior modification of obesity has been paralleled by an enormous increase of interest on the part of the lay public. Research results have found their way with increasing frequency into the popular press, and treatment programs based upon behavioral principles are consistently over-subscribed. The demand for help in the control of obesity has even led to the recent publication of self-help manuals based upon behavioral principles and presented in the form of programmed texts.

In this climate of high expectations and limited treatment resources, the program developed by Dr. Ferguson may be particularly useful. It is based upon a sound background of research, tempered by intensive clinical testing designed to refine and polish the most effective techniques and to ascertain the optimal order of their presentation. During the past several months I have had occasion to use Dr. Ferguson's program and have found it very well-suited to the treatment of the majority of obese people who have come to the Stanford Eating Disorders Clinic.

The program is particularly effective in its presentation of techniques which fall into the general category of stimulus control. Many of these techniques are a matter of common sense and have been in common use in weight reduction efforts in the past: for example, developing the automatic habit of making low-calorie foods like celery and raw carrots readily available. Persons who have used such techniques in the past are thereby encouraged to try them again while newcomers are exposed to these time-tested maneuvers. Other techniques may be new to overweight persons. A particularly effective one, developed from theories on stimulus control, is the establishment of a "designated eating place," where all food, meals and snacks alike, are to be consumed.

A key feature of any behavior modification program, and one which is particularly well exemplified in Dr. Ferguson's program, is the use of feedback about performance. A cornerstone of behavioral programs has been the use of a Food Diary to help people become aware of what they eat and the circumstances under which they eat. They are invaluable in helping people to define problem times, places and circumstances of over-eating. They may even by themselves reduce eating; at times it is simpler not to eat than to have to write down what one has eaten.

This program contains a number of innovative forms of feedback beyond the Food Diary. The "Eating Place Record" provides useful information about the extent to which the person is achieving the goal of confining all eating to the "designated eating place." The "Behavioral Analysis Form" depicts progress made in cutting down on snacking and confining eating to mealtimes. The use of "an eating ratio" provides feedback on the rate of eating, valuable information in helping to reduce its speed.

A deceptively simple form of feedback is built into one of the most effective behavioral control measures in the program. This is pre-planning of meals and snacks. Writing down exactly what will be eaten during one or more meals on the following day provides strong incentives to eat these foods and to resist impulse eating. Pre-planned foods are written in one color of ink, the actual foods consumed in another. The decreasing amount of two-colored Diary pages is a reassuring reminder of progress to date and problems to be overcome.

Many of the techniques utilized in this and other behavioral programs for obesity are standard ones based upon problems which are found among most overweight people. Each person, however, has problems which are specific to him, and Dr. Ferguson's program provides guidance in identifying such problems and in coping with them. Such problem-solving exercises are among the most attractive features of this program. . . .

Behavioral modification is no panacea. It demands of participants a great deal of hard work and often major changes in personal habits and life situations. But for those who succeed, the results are well worth the effort. For behavioral programs can lead not only to the control of obesity, but also to a more rewarding inner-directed life.

Albert J. Stunkard, M.D.

ACKNOWLEDGEMENTS

The work of many scientists has contributed to the preparation of this manual. Techniques have been incorporated from a wide variety of sources--psychology, psychiatry, medicine, physiology, and common sense. Although many of the individual investigators in the field of appetite and weight control are mentioned in the bibliography, there are countless others who have made significant contributions to the body of information from which this text has been developed. Without this basic research carried out by hundreds of individuals working in many scientific disciplines, there would be no hope for an effective control of obesity.

I would like to specifically express my gratitude to two great teachers and friends, Dr. Albert J. Stunkard and Dr. W. Stewart Agras. Without their help, encouragement, and continued interest, this book would probably not have been started and certainly would have never been finished.

The clinical program from which this text evolved was repeatedly tested and revised at the Stanford Eating Disorders Clinic in the Department of Psychiatry and Behavioral Sciences at Stanford Medical School and the La Jolla Eating Disorders Clinic in La Jolla, California. Evaluation groups were conducted and the program critiqued by a number of friends, many of whom are now widely dispersed from Stanford. These include: Billie Bem, M.S.W., Children's Hospital, San Francisco; Stan Chapman, Ph.D., Emory University; Carlos C. Greaves, M.D., Centro Medico Docente La Trinidad, Caracas, Venezuela; Brandon Qualls, M.D., Brown University; Colleen Rand, Ph.D., Stanford University; Jan Ruby, Stanford University; C.B. Taylor, M.D., Stanford University; Roger Walsh, M.D., Ph.D., Stanford University; Joellen Werene, M.D., Stanford University, Carolyn Wright, B.A., University of California San Diego

Medical School and Eileen Riordan, R.D. in La Jolla. I want to express my appreciation to each of them for their critical feedback and many words of encouragement when they were sorely needed.

The patients who used the program at Stanford contributed immeasurably to its development. Their participation ranged from the reinforcement I felt when they lost weight to their many helpful suggestions about format and style.

Encouragement for this revision has come from colleagues across the continent. Dr. Stunkard at the University of Pennsylvania, Mr. Milt Miles with Nestle Enterprises in Cleveland, and John Munro in Scotland have been quite effective with their gentle pressure to complete the chapters which were started ten years ago. A final thanks goes to Dave Bull, who has patiently guided me through the maze of publication, and to my wife and children who have waited for me at home on those many evenings when I have been at the clinic teaching people to change their eating habits.

LESSON ONE
INTRODUCTION TO THE BEHAVIORAL CONTROL OF WEIGHT—
HABIT AWARENESS

INTRODUCTION TO THE PROGRAM

You are beginning this behavioral program to learn how to control your weight. During the next 21 weeks you will work to change your eating and exercise habits, and many of the attitudes and self defeating thoughts that have "helped" you become overweight or have sabotaged your success in the past. Your weight, which brought you to this program, will be one of the ways you measure how effective you are at changing your eating habits. The more they change and the more you are able to control your eating behaviors, the more weight you will lose.

Weigh-in

Weigh yourself and record your weight on the Personal Weight Record located on page 323 . Since this is the first piece of information on the Weight Record, it is important that you put it in the correct place on the form. Today there will be no weight change to calculate. The large dot at the top of the diagonal line on the graph paper indicates the starting point for your weight graph.

Today you will begin by weighing yourself and recording your weight on the Personal Weight Record. Each week you will repeat this process, as close to the same time of day as possible. Next week you will add the additional step of calculating and graphing your weight change. (In subsequent weeks you will calculate first your weight change during the week, then your cumulative weight change since the beginning of the program.) This will help you see exactly how well your weight change program is progressing each week.

The solid diagonal line across the graph on your Personal Weight Record shows a weight loss of one pound a week. The areas enclosed by the slashed diagonal lines on both sides of the solid line show the amount of change for faster losers (2 lbs. per week) and slower losers (1/2 lb. per week).

You may lose faster or more slowly, and your rate of loss may change from week to week. Everyone loses at a different rate! The solid diagonal line will keep reminding you of how your rate of weight loss compares with the one-pound-per-week rate. Figure 1 shows how a complete weight graph looks for several individuals in a behavioral weight control group.

Each lesson begins with a weighing, then homework correction, a review, and then a new lesson. The homework is designed to be completed in one-week blocks. To use the program most effectively, *you should not go faster* than one lesson each week. Even though these lessons appear simple, they call for important changes—trying to speed up almost always leads to failure.

A reward system has been built into the program to help you stay motivated to finish all twenty-one lessons and to do all of the homework. Set aside some money today, say, one hundred dollars, for a personal reward. (The $100 is not a magic figure; it should be an amount that you can afford, but which is meaningful for you. There is no reason why you or someone else can't "up the ante," if you feel you want to work for higher stakes.) It should be separated from other funds: not "... there in the household budget when I need it." Ideally, it should be removed from your control. Lock it away, or give it to someone else to hold for you. This is *your* reward money.

At the end of the book you will find a Homework Credit Sheet which shows the refund value of each piece of homework (based on a reward of $100). For each lesson you will be asked to complete all of the homework, even when you may feel that you don't need it or feel that it is busy work. For credit, all that counts is that you have done the homework. There are no right or wrong answers. Give yourself full credit towards a refund if you complete the homework forms each week.

FIGURE 1. WEEKLY WEIGHT LOSS FOR INDIVIDUAL MEMBERS OF A BEHAVIORAL WEIGHT CONTROL GROUP

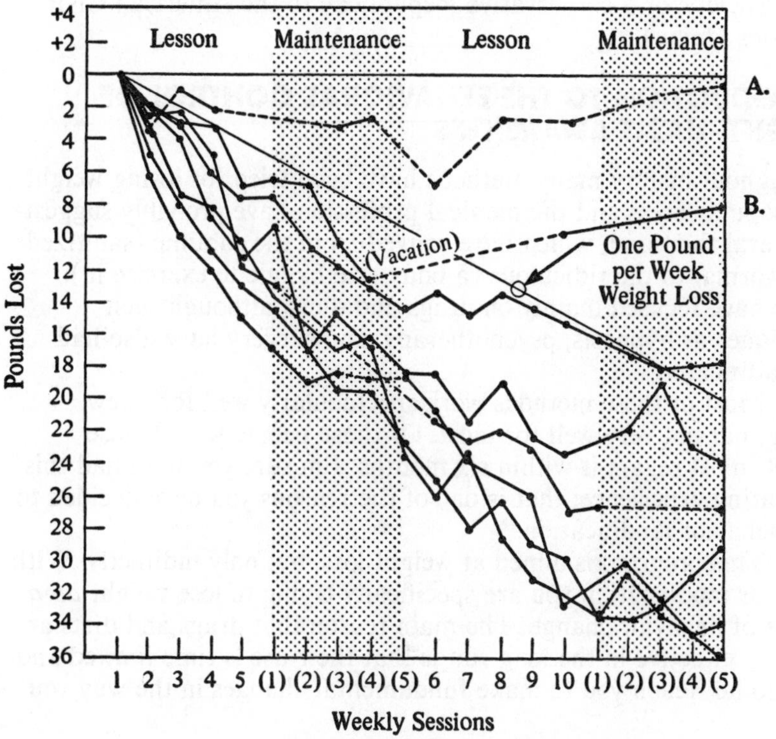

Each group member is represented by one line. Broken lines indicate missed meetings, shaded areas represent Maintenance weeks. Patient A was a businessman who could not attend meetings regularly; Patient B went on vacation during the second half of the course.

At the end of 21 weeks you will total up the amount of credit you have earned, and then pay yourself that amount of money out of your reward fund. It is yours to spend as you see fit, preferably on yourself. Any extra unearned amount should be given away—to a worthy cause, or even more motivating, to a cause you do not believe in (for example, a liberal Democrat making a donation to the John Birch Society, or a conservative Republican to the American Civil Liberties Union).

INTRODUCTION TO THE BEHAVIORAL CONTROL OF WEIGHT–HABIT AWARENESS

Throughout history many methods have been tried for losing weight. The popular press and the medical profession have probably suggested several thousand, which have ranged from the sublime (sanitized tape worms) to the ridiculous (a body-size baggie to exercise in). These have focused mainly on drugs and diets, although such techniques as hypnosis, psychotherapy, and surgery have also had their advocates.

Most of these methods work spectacularly well for a few people, but not very well for most. Of those people who do lose weight, most regain it within six months. I'm sure you have had this frustrating experience; that is one of the reasons you have decided to try "behavior modification."

This program is aimed at weight loss, but only indirectly. With behavior modification you are specifically trying to lose weight *as a result* of behavior change. The main reason that drugs and diets are not very effective in the long run is that their use is time limited and they do not teach you to make fundamental changes in the way you eat.

When a drug or diet treatment program is over, most people resume their old patterns of eating and regain their weight. This is especially true for individuals in stressful situations, or people with chaotic life styles.

Regaining weight does not mean that they are weak-willed, or not trying. However, while they were losing weight they did not learn to eat and exercise in a more sensible manner; their eating and exercise habits did not change, and when they found themselves back in the real world with real food, they simply ate in the same way they had always eaten in the past, and they resumed their sedentary life style.

The object of this program is to teach you to be active, and to eat in a way that will lead to weight loss and permanent weight control. Although it may take more of your time than a series of shots or pills, and in many ways is more demanding than a diet, there are real advantages to this method. A follow-up survey of patients in a University of Pennsylvania program showed that of those who lost 20 or more pounds (over 50 percent of the original group), more than 80 percent were able to keep that weight off for over two years. (1)

It is impossible to make any promises as to the outcome of this program. It will depend entirely on you. Some people do extremely well; others never become fully engaged in the program, or are unwilling or unable to put the time and effort into the individual lessons, and as a consequence, they do not lose as much weight.

Weight loss is important for your morale, and it is an indicator of how much progress you are making; but once again, the primary goal of *Habits Not Diets* is behavior change—not weight loss.

On the other hand, you are reading this book because you are ultimately interested in weight loss, and you should be optimistic about your chances of long-term success. Used with groups, this program has resulted in an average loss of about 1 pound per week for each group member. Many people are able to lose twice this fast. Many never regain it!

The control of eating and activity habits (and consequent weight loss) is largely a matter of establishing priorities. If it is not important for you to lose weight, you won't. If you do not set aside the time to do the program, to change your habits, you will fail.

To follow this program and to be successful takes time and effort and commitment. You will be expected to take more time eating than you do now, to experience food more thoroughly, and to enjoy everything you eat. I want you to become active—not a world class athlete, but at least active enough to elevate your metabolism, and to burn off some calories. If you cannot spare the time to really eat, and get some meaningful exercise, your program will probably be unsuccessful.

Theories About Obesity

There are many theories explaining why people become obese, some of which apply to only a few individuals. For most people who are overweight, the cause is unknown. In 99 percent of the cases, exhaustive medical tests and investigation will be negative; no specific cause will be found for the weight problem. Only in few cases can the cause of obesity be identified. These have included thyroid, pituitary, or adrenal malfunction, varieties of diabetes, rare tumors, and very uncommon neurological disorders.

There are also general factors like the tendency of everyone to put on weight as he or she grows older. Unfortunately, caloric needs decrease with age at the same time in life that we become more sedentary (and often tend to take the elevator more often and eat more luxurious meals).

Finally, there are inherited tendencies to be overweight. This factor is difficult to separate from environmental learning because eating habits tend to be very similar among members of the same family: We eat like our parents ate, both with regard to style of eating, and in our food preferences and cooking methods.

Many therapists still adhere to personality trait theories and believe that overweight individuals have deep-seated psychological problems which are compensated for by eating, or emotional states which are represented by an "equivalent in eating behaviors." Research has shown that individuals with "deep-seated psychological problems" rarely lose weight with traditional psychiatric or psychological treatments, despite greater insight into their problems. Their problems are probably not the cause of their obesity.

Finally, there is the theory that individuals who became obese when they were young acquired too many fat cells as a result of overeating in early childhood. There is some evidence for this theory, and it can be a relative handicap for anyone fighting weight problems. However, it does not make weight loss impossible. In outcome studies, total weight loss has been found to be comparable, where groups of patients with childhood onset obesity were compared with groups who became obese as adults. The amount lost was the same, regardless of when the extra weight was gained.

The ultimate cause of obesity is more energy taken into your body than is used. The excess is stored as fat. If this imbalance can be corrected, if you become able to take in fewer calories than you burn up each day, your overweight problem will be corrected, regardless of its cause.

(At this point, and regularly throughout this book, you will be asked to pause and reflect—and to re-read parts you find are unclear.)

Is Everything Clear?

- Do you see why it is necessary to learn new behaviors to keep weight off? Yes _______ No _______

- What goes wrong with diets, pills, and other weight control methods?

  1. ____

2. ______________________________

Over-eating and inactivity are behavior patterns that have been learned and practiced for years. Like all firmly entrenched habits, they continue because they pay off.

Relief of hunger is one of the most obvious rewards for eating; but I think that after reflecting a bit you will be able to think of many situations in which you eat which are not related to hunger. For example, many people eat in response to anxiety, anger, happiness, frustration, sadness, fatigue, insomnia, social pressure, and boredom.

Because there are so many influences on your eating habits, because you have *learned* to eat in response to so many situations, these eating behaviors are very hard to change. It takes a thorough and systematic program of working on almost every aspect of your life to free you from all the stimuli that tell you to eat.

Take a minute and list four situations or feelings that might start you eating—that are not directly related to sitting down at a regular meal.

1. ______________________________

2. ______________________________

3. ______________________________

4. ______________________________

As you can see, there are many reasons to eat beyond hunger. Most of them are learned—that is, you have learned that food makes boredom or frustration or other unpleasant situations easier to tolerate.

Learning New Eating Behaviors

Thinking of eating behaviors as learned is an optimistic way to look at the problem of being overweight. If you have excess pounds because of learned habits, then the solution seems obvious —you have to learn a new set of behaviors to take the place of the old ones. You have to eat in a new way. It may be necessary to pursue this retraining to the point of actually learning a new way of putting your food in your mouth! As you establish new eating habits, almost automatically the old patterns which are no longer practiced will gradually fade away.

It is very important to understand that the goals of this program are not to stop eating, or simply to diet, but to develop a new set of eating and activity habits, so that when you lose weight, it stays off. This involves not only the type and amount of food you choose to eat, but also how, when, where, and with whom you eat, and the circumstances under which you acquire food.

In this program the focus will be on strengthening "good" eating habits rather than trying to weaken "bad" ones. The reason for this is simple: It is easier to learn a new habit than to try to forget an old one. Furthermore, if you can make the new habit incompatible with the old one, the old habit will naturally decrease in strength, since the two cannot happen at the same time. For example, it is impossible to "wolf" down a meal in a few minutes if you put your fork down after each bite.

One of the first things you will do in this program is to develop *habit awareness*. You will examine in detail your present eating habits and determine the specific behaviors that have contributed to your present weight problem. Once you have identified these behaviors, you will proceed to figure out which environmental conditions control them. Finally, you will be in a position to make changes in your environment which will encourage the new behaviors that you are striving for.

Changing any habit—smoking, drinking, or eating—is very hard, especially if you try to do it all at once. The way around the difficulty is to break down the behavior you want to change into its simpler parts (for example, shopping, preparing food, and identification of where and when you eat) and to work on each part, one at a time. This makes the going slow, but when you begin to feel that things are too slow, remember how many years it took your present way of eating to evolve, and how much faster (albeit over several months) this program will be.

You are trying to reverse, and to develop substitute behaviors for some of the strongest habit patterns in your daily life. To try to change them overnight would only invite failure. The way to succeed is to take small steps and to practice each one until it is "over learned," until it seems second nature, until it is a new habit.

Some weeks in this program, you will be presented techniques for altering your eating environment which you will be able to learn and master readily. Other weeks the lesson may introduce a behavioral control technique that is difficult for you. This is inevitable. If necessary, take a couple of weeks extra to master any step that seems especially difficult for you—don't try to go too fast or jump ahead. You will only be courting failure.

Try not to place pressure on yourself by saying "this is so

simple a three-year-old could do it." What seems simple on paper—like eating each meal only at an appropriate place—is often very difficult and complicated in practice. (Of course you are right—a three-year-old could do it—they've never done it another way.)

Changing behaviors takes time, and your weight loss in this twenty-one week program may not be what you hoped for at the beginning. I can sympathize with this and wish there were a magic way to produce changes—there isn't. It takes time and a lot of effort to change, and at this point the last thing you need is moralizing about being overweight—to put the book down, to feel guilty, and perhaps to say, "to hell with it."

You may not be able to master some of the techniques. That's O.K. There is no race and no competition. The object is not to make you feel bad, but to help you control the stimuli that cause you to over-eat. Although nothing would be lost by going on a sensible diet while you are involved in this program (you would learn just as much about behavior control and you would probably lose weight faster), the choice of whether to include a diet is yours. The program does *not* include a diet; the purpose is to learn to eat *anything*—with control.

However, if you do decide to diet, it should be moderate—1000-1200 calories per day for women and 1200-1500 calories per day for men—so you have eating behaviors and habits to work with and to change. There aren't very many significant eating behaviors to modify in the vacuum of a 600-calorie-a-day eggplant and grapefruit diet.

Weight loss is *not* a behavior. You have begun this program to change your eating behaviors, and you should not judge your progress solely by weight loss. As you know, weight loss can occur for a variety of reasons. In most weight loss programs, with weight loss as the sole criterion for success, people are subtly encouraged to do anything to lose weight before they weigh in. They starve themselves for the day, or use laxatives or diuretics before they are weighed.

You should strive for weight loss as a result of changed eating habits. Each week you will check your weight and at the same time you will be grading your homework as a way of checking your progress with your eating behaviors. Ultimately you will be your own weight control expert, and you will monitor your eating habits automatically. Weight will become a secondary concern. The value of the educational approach we will be using is that once you have learned the principles and techniques of self- management, you will be able to apply them to all of the situations to which you are exposed. There will be no more going on and off of diets.

By learning new eating habits and losing weight you will find that people react to you differently, that your self-image will change, and that you will enjoy eating more. Every pattern of behavior has its consequences. Over-eating leads to a change in body size, a poor self-image, and a loss of mobility. This, in turn, leads to a loss of self-esteem, and often depression.

Changing eating patterns can affect many aspects of your life, and you can expect to have different experiences in the world. These experiences, for example, being accepted by others and being admired, can in turn lead you to change your way of thinking and feeling about yourself—and eventually to a greater control of your eating.

As you lose weight, expect changes to take place in other areas of your life. If you are threatened by looking thin, by looking sexier, by looking more athletic, and by receiving compliments about these types of attributes, think twice about losing weight. If you are not bothered by these thoughts, enjoy the changes.

The rewards for weight loss are not immediate. It takes time for the health, appearance, and social benefits to accumulate. On the other hand, eating provides an immediate reward, which sometimes makes it difficult to remember the long-term benefits of not eating, until it is too late. By taking small steps, adding small behavior changes each week, it is possible to change. Eating skills, like any other skills, take time to develop and perfect.

You have total responsibility for yourself in this program. Although you want to lose weight, to do so you have to be willing to make some difficult changes in your eating habits. Some of these changes, such as putting your fork down between bites, may seem silly in a social context. To solve this conflict you have to assign priorities to your behaviors and try to avoid the trap of saying, "That's a good idea, but I could never do it because...." When this happens, you have to ask yourself, "What are my priorities?" For example, is not being able to spend time eating breakfast more important than losing weight?

There are no right and wrong answers, and at some point behavior change and weight reduction may not be as high on your list of priorities as other behaviors, such as getting to work early, or taking only five minutes for lunch between assignments.

Weight reduction is not easy, but it doesn't have to be a painful, or even a hungry experience. It is a long-term project, and it will be successful only on that basis. Short-term gains and losses are relatively unimportant.

To make this program work, it is important that you understand the principles, both now at the start, and when new ideas are introduced. But even when you understand each technique, and are satisfied that you can apply that technique to your life, your work is not finished. It is essential that you *practice*, until these techniques become habits.

For many people, the most difficult aspect of this program is the necessary repetitiveness. It is a system based on repetition, which necessarily emphasizes points over and over, and encourages you to practice the techniques frequently. Don't get discouraged when you feel a point has been made more often than you would like—that's what makes this program work!

Part of every behavior change program is the concept of measurement. You need to know where you stand with your current behaviors, to know whether or not the behavior changes you have introduced have been effective.

The period of observation before any changes are introduced is called "the baseline." During this time you collect information about a particular habit or set of behaviors that you want to change or modify. When you have become aware of your eating habits, during a week of baseline observation, you will be able to see eating patterns that can be easily changed. The following week's observation will tell you if you have been successful in modifying the behaviors you identified during the baseline period.

The Food Diary

In this program a great deal of emphasis is placed on keeping records of eating behaviors and activity patterns, both to tell you what you are doing now, and to enable you to see when a change has occurred. The first record you will be keeping is a daily food diary. The purpose of this record is habit awareness: to make you aware of how you eat and to gather baseline information about your eating habits.

One of the first things you will notice during the coming weeks is that accurately keeping the diary will make you very aware of everything you eat. The natural tendency will be to decrease the amount of food you eat. You will start to question yourself each time you begin to eat, and to question the need for each food portion you are considering eating.

One of the benefits of this increased awareness will be a delay between impulse and action—you will stop and think. Initially this may be more in the form of, "I don't want to write this down, it's too much work and easier just not to eat it." Eventually this type of internal dialogue will change to something more like, "I really don't want to eat that; I'm not hungry now."

The food diary has several columns which ask you to report on different behaviors and feelings. The column headings will change from week to week as the emphases of the lessons change; however, a food diary in some form will be part of each lesson.

Let's Review a Bit

- Do you understand the theory of behavior change?
  Yes ______ No ______ (If you answered No, re-read this lesson.)

- Do you see why this is a slow program? Yes ______ No ______

- Why does it have to be slow—why take small steps?

  ____

  (To insure success.)

- Why are self-observation and homework so important?

  ____

  (Homework and self-observation are the only ways you have of assessing behavior change; you cannot measure eating behaviors directly. Even your weight each week is only an indirect measure of changed behavior.)

- Do you understand why behavior change and weight loss have to be high priority items in your life if this program is going to work?

  ____

  (Because you will be tempted to give up, or to pick and choose techniques.)

HOMEWORK

Among the materials for today's lesson you will find a sample of a filled-in food diary and seven blank food diary forms. They are divided horizontally by lines that represent 6:00 a.m., 11:00 a.m., 4:00 p.m., and 9:00 p.m. These lines separate your eating into four time categories (the 3 customary meal times, and an added snack time).

In the first vertical column you record the actual starting time for each meal or snack. In the next column, mark down the length in minutes of each such meal or snack. Mark an "M" or "S" in the third column, depending on whether it is a meal or snack, and rate that eating episode on a scale of 0 to 4 in the "H" column to indicate the degree of your hunger: "0" indicates no hunger, or the feeling you have after a large meal; "1" is some hunger; "2" is normal hunger; "3" is a good healthy hunger; and "4" is equivalent to the hungriest you have ever been.

Describe your body position by a number code: "1"— walking, "2"—standing, "3"—sitting, "4"—lying down. In the "Activity" column, indicate activities carried out while eating; for example, watching television, reading the paper, or working. "Location of Eating" asks for a short description of where you eat the meal or snack; for example, "car," "desk," "kitchen table." In the "Kind of Food" column, indicate the content of your meal or snack.

For this exercise, the quantity of food is not as important as the type of food—so that next week you can answer the question: How many times did I eat high-calorie food when I wasn't hungry?

Save your completed food diaries. The information on them will be used in future lessons.

The second form for this week's homework is a sheet of graph paper. Draw a rough plan of your house on this piece of paper. (A filled-in sample form is included in the homework section of this chapter in front of the blank form you will fill out at home.) Precision is not as important as completeness in including such food-related objects as your television set, desk, telephone, table, refrigerator, etc.

During the next week, put a small "M" or "S" at the appropriate places on the plan to mark where you eat each meal or snack. This will give you a picture of how random or spread out your eating places are at home. If you want to involve the family, or feel that their eating or snacking behaviors influence you, you can suggest that they mark the same graph with a different color. In this way, you can make a map for the whole family's eating pattern for a week.

Finally, the day before you read the next chapter, go through the house and look for food—any food. Mark with an "X" on your floor plan each "find"—even a few pieces of candy by the TV or a candy bar hidden in the closet.

Each week you will have homework similar to today's. You will check your homework next week and record whether or not it was completed on your Homework Credit schedule. Each week you will credit a portion of your (let's assume $100) homework deposit to yourself for each part of the homework assignment completed. This small amount of money credited each week often makes the difference between carrying out assignments and forgetting to do them. It is a really good feeling to finish the program both 20 pounds lighter and 100 dollars richer.

A final suggestion to help increase the probability of success: Involve someone else in your behavior change program. Teach your lessons to your spouse, children, neighbors, co-workers, schoolmates, or anyone you see regularly. This will not only help them understand what you are going through, but it will also give you a chance to solidify your learning when you put all of the instructional materials into your own words to teach someone else. Most people are eager to be included. Soon you may find you have started a class of your own. Teaching others can only benefit your own personal weight control program.

In summary, most eating patterns are learned behaviors. The way to control weight and maintain weight loss is not through dieting. This program is not a diet, it is a method of controlling your environment and the stimuli that cause you to eat in a way that results in weight loss. By systematically applying a wide variety of behavior change techniques, it is possible to learn new patterns of eating behaviors. These changes must be introduced a small step at a time.

In many ways changing eating habits is like playing the piano. To expect anything more than scales and exercises at first would be silly. By the end of this course, we hope to have you playing Mozart.

Consider What You Have Read

- If you have a question about any aspect of the homework, the food diary, or the house plan, re-read the relevant part of the text. It is very important that you understand each step as you go along.

The homework assignment for this week is:

A. Complete Lesson One Food Diary.

B. Record the location of all eating episodes on house plan.

C. Locate food throughout house and record its location on the house plan.

INSTRUCTIONS FOR FILLING OUT THE FOOD DIARY—Week One

Time: starting time for a meal or snack

Minutes Spent Eating: length of eating episode in minutes

M/S: indicate type of eating by the appropriate letter, "M" = meal or "S" = snack.

H: hunger on a scale of 0 to 4. 0 = no hunger, 4 = extreme hunger

Body Position: 1—walking
2—standing
3—sitting
4—lying down

Activity While Eating: Record any activity you carry out while eating, such as watching television, reading, or sweeping the floor.

Location of Eating: Record each place you eat; for example your car, kitchen table, or living room couch.

Kind of Food: Indicate the content of your meal or snack by kind of food.

Sample

FOOD DIARY — Lesson One

Day of Week Monday Date

Time	Minutes Spent Eating	M/S	H	BP	Activity While Eating	Location of Eating	Kind of Food
6:00							
7:20-7:30	10 min	M	0	3	Paper	Kitchen	Coffee Cereal
8:15-8:20	5 min	S	0	2	Talking	Work	Donut Coffee
10:30-?	5 min	S	1	1	Walking	Hall	Donut
11:00							
12:30	1 min	S	2	2	Work	Desk	Candy Bar
3:30–3:40	10 min	M	3	3	Reading	Restaurant	Hamburger
4:00							
5:30-6	½ hr	S	3	3	Paper/TV	L.R.	Scotch/water nuts
6-7	1 hr	M	2	3	TV	D.R.	Beef TV Dinner Ice Cream
9:00							
10:30–10:45	15 min	S	0	2	TV	LR	Ice Cream

M/S: Meal or Snack; H: Degree of Hunger (0 = None, 1 = Some, 2 = Normal, 3 = Good Healthy Hunger, 4 = Ravenous); BP: Body Position: 1 = Walking, 2 = Standing, 3 = Sitting, 4 = Lying Down

FOOD DIARY — Lesson One

Day of Week ____________________ Date ____________________

Time	Minutes Spent Eating	M/S	H	BP	Activity While Eating	Location of Eating	Kind of Food
6:00							
11:00							
4:00							
9:00							

M/S: Meal or Snack; H: Degree of Hunger (0 = None, 1 = Some, 2 = Normal, 3 = Good Healthy Hunger, 4 = Ravenous); BP: Body Position: 1 = Walking, 2 = Standing, 3 = Sitting, 4 = Lying Down

FOOD DIARY — Lesson One

Day of Week ____________________ Date ____________________

Time	Minutes Spent Eating	M/S	H	BP	Activity While Eating	Location of Eating	Kind of Food
6:00							
11:00							
4:00							
9:00							

M/S: Meal or Snack; H: Degree of Hunger (0 = None, 1 = Some, 2 = Normal, 3 = Good Healthy Hunger, 4 = Ravenous); BP: Body Position: 1 = Walking, 2 = Standing, 3 = Sitting, 4 = Lying Down

FOOD DIARY — Lesson One

Day of Week ______________________ Date ______________________

Time	Minutes Spent Eating	M/S	H	BP	Activity While Eating	Location of Eating	Kind of Food
6:00							
11:00							
4:00							
9:00							

M/S: Meal or Snack; H: Degree of Hunger (0 = None, 1 = Some, 2 = Normal, 3 = Good Healthy Hunger, 4 = Ravenous); BP: Body Position: 1 = Walking, 2 = Standing, 3 = Sitting, 4 = Lying Down

FOOD DIARY — Lesson One

Day of Week ____________________ Date ____________________

Time	Minutes Spent Eating	M/S	H	BP	Activity While Eating	Location of Eating	Kind of Food
6:00							
11:00							
4:00							
9:00							

M/S: Meal or Snack; H: Degree of Hunger (0 = None, 1 = Some, 2 = Normal, 3 = Good Healthy Hunger, 4 = Ravenous); BP: Body Position: 1 = Walking, 2 = Standing, 3 = Sitting, 4 = Lying Down

FOOD DIARY — Lesson One

Day of Week ____________________ Date ____________________

Time	Minutes Spent Eating	M/S	H	BP	Activity While Eating	Location of Eating	Kind of Food
6:00							
11:00							
4:00							
9:00							

M/S: Meal or Snack; H: Degree of Hunger (0 = None, 1 = Some, 2 = Normal, 3 = Good Healthy Hunger, 4 = Ravenous); BP: Body Position: 1 = Walking, 2 = Standing, 3 = Sitting, 4 = Lying Down

FOOD DIARY — Lesson One

Day of Week ______________________ Date ______________________

Time	Minutes Spent Eating	M/S	H	BP	Activity While Eating	Location of Eating	Kind of Food
6:00							
11:00							
4:00							
9:00							

M/S: Meal or Snack; H: Degree of Hunger (0 = None, 1 = Some, 2 = Normal, 3 = Good Healthy Hunger, 4 = Ravenous); BP: Body Position: 1 = Walking, 2 = Standing, 3 = Sitting, 4 = Lying Down

FOOD DIARY — Lesson One

Day of Week ____________________ Date ____________________

Time	Minutes Spent Eating	M/S	H	BP	Activity While Eating	Location of Eating	Kind of Food
6:00							
11:00							
4:00							
9:00							

M/S: Meal or Snack; H: Degree of Hunger (0 = None, 1 = Some, 2 = Normal, 3 = Good Healthy Hunger, 4 = Ravenous); BP: Body Position: 1 = Walking, 2 = Standing, 3 = Sitting, 4 = Lying Down

SAMPLE

HOUSE PLAN

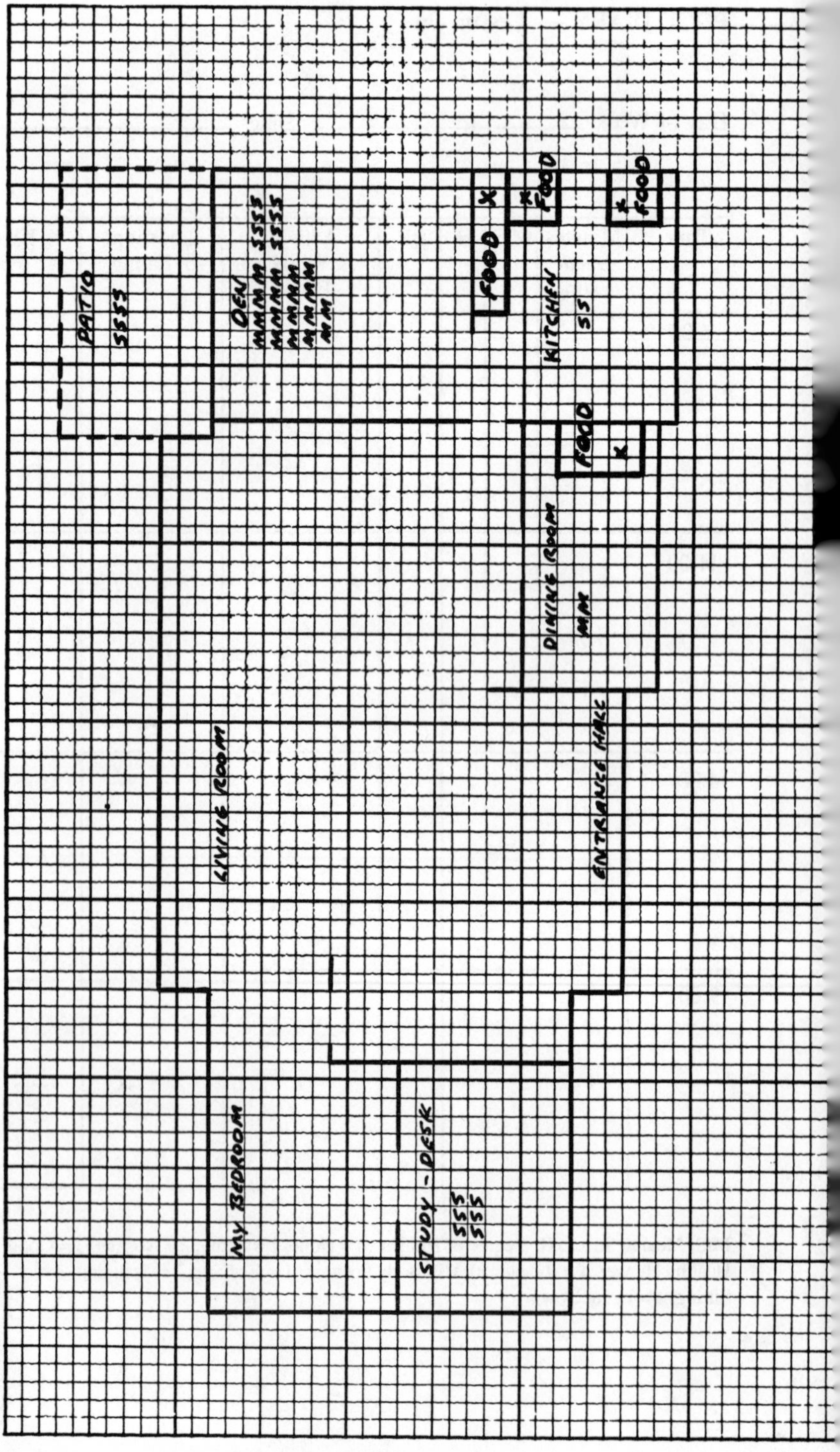

HOUSE PLAN

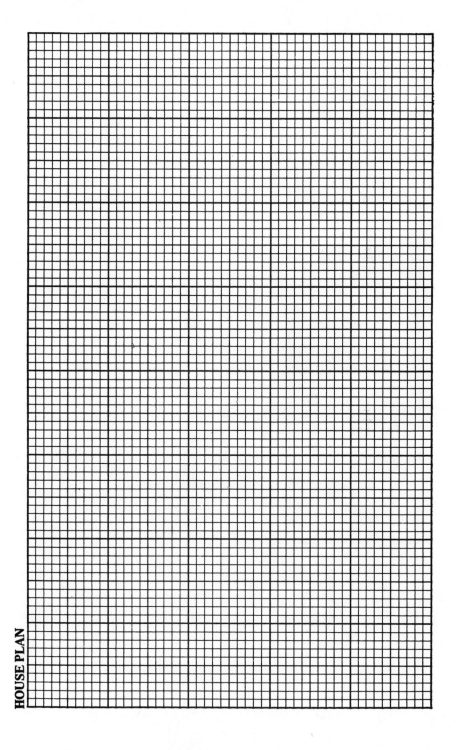

LESSON TWO

HOME DECALORIZATION—WHAT YOU DON'T HAVE, YOU WON'T EAT

WEIGH-IN AND HOMEWORK

Weigh yourself and record your weight on your Personal Weight Record at the end of the book. Fill in your weight change since the first lesson. (Subtract today's weight from last week's weight.) Place this figure in the boxes labeled "Weight Change" and "Total Weight Change." Make a mark on the line on the Personal Weight Record graph labeled "Week Two" to indicate the weight change for the past week. To graph your weight change, connect that mark with the dot on the line labeled "Week One."

This procedure will be repeated each week, with your weight, change of weight, and graphed difference recorded on your Personal Weight Record.

Check your homework for Lesson One.

- Lesson One Food Diary complete? Yes ______ No ______
- House Plan? Yes ______ No ______

Briefly read back over your diaries for each day and check to see if you completed them. If you had any problems filling them out, refer back to the initial instructions.

In addition, see if you can identify any unusual eating patterns, things to work on during the program (like always standing up while eating snacks, eating while speeding to work on the freeway, or eating pizza six times a week). Do not make a detailed analysis of the food items or patterns of behavior. We will come back to this in a later lesson.

Check the house plan to make sure it has been completed. Indicate which portions of the homework you have completed, by initialling the appropriate square on the Homework Credit schedule. This will count toward the amount of money you will have earned at the end of the program as a reward for completing the homework.

REVIEW

Much of our behavior is unconscious and automatic. If someone asks you what you were feeling when you ate lunch yesterday, where you were when you had your mid-afternoon snack 2 days ago, with whom you were eating breakfast a week ago last Wednesday, or what time it was when you had dinner on Tuesday, you probably would not know the answer.

This type of information is *not* usually stored in our consciousness, and is therefore unavailable when we want to use the information as part of a behavior change program. It is precisely these types of connections between time of day, feeling state, place, and social environment that are important in modifying eating behaviors. Written records are one way to make sure this information isn't lost, so that subsequently it can be analyzed, dissected, and used. It provides information for a baseline, or knowing where you started from, and information later on to show you how much you've changed.

The overall strategy for self-monitoring is simple. Determine what it is you want to observe, and when it occurs, and write it down promptly. For example, in the food diary last week, you wrote down a number of things associated with eating that ranged from how hungry you were to where you were eating.

Many people will be amazed at how little hunger they experience with many of their eating episodes during the day. A written food diary also helps the "nibbler," or the person who snacks frequently. It's quite enlightening to look at a food diary and realize that there are 20 episodes per day of eating, when you thought you were only eating 3 regular meals a day and a snack here and there. It's not that you are lying to yourself, it is simply that this type of information is not stored in your memory.

This is a behavior modification program. You are learning self-management techniques to change and control your eating behaviors and activity patterns. The ultimate goal of this course is to apply these techniques to your life in such a way that you lose weight.

Weight loss *per se* is not the main objective at this point. You should lose weight, but as a result of behavior change. One of the basic points stressed in Lesson One was that this is *not* a program designed to increase "will power." If you learn new eating habits, the strength of old ones will slowly decrease. There will be no need to struggle with "will power." Your task is not to stop eating, but to eat differently.

Changing behaviors, especially those as ingrained as eating and exercise behaviors, takes time. Years of practice have formed these habits and they are often immediately rewarding. As a result, they cannot be unlearned overnight. This lesson introduced a general principle of behavior modification and showed you how to apply it to specific behaviors.

The techniques may sound tedious, or too simple, or too compulsive, or too difficult, or any number of things, but we have found that approaching these longstanding habits slowly and methodically, a step at a time, works best. These techniques have the historical advantage of working for most people who use them.

This approach to the problem of obesity is quite different from traditional psychotherapy. You probably will not gain insight into the possible psychological reasons for your excess weight, nor will you achieve dramatic solutions to any deep personal problems. That's not the point; the object of these lessons is simply to help you learn new eating skills.

Be on the lookout for a couple of common problems, which you may run into during the program: The tendency to feel or say, "I am fat and will never be able to change," a "what the hell" attitude that will clearly defeat you; or, "That's a good idea, but I couldn't possibly do it because...," a self-defeating pattern of rejecting help that will also lead to failure.

Weight loss is a matter of arranging priorities in your life. Your eating habits mesh with your social life, work and recreation. It is hard to change part of the system without an effect on the other parts. Again, one reason we will start slowly in changing behaviors is because it is difficult to change deeply-rooted patterns that interlock with many other behaviors.

The way to learn new habits is through a series of exercises that you can approach creatively. Use that spark of brilliance inside yourself to make it work!

Remember also, that the more you can involve others—your

family, friends, people at work, or even total strangers—the better your chances of success. Don't be afraid to tell them you are doing something new. If you can get the people around you to help keep track of your behaviors, to help prompt or cue you, it will be much easier to change.

This weight control program should be a serious undertaking—your willingness to read this book indicates that kind of commitment. It can be an enjoyable experience, and if taken a step at a time, it is not difficult. Even climbing a mountain like Everest can be broken into single simple steps taken one at a time. Like mountain climbing, if you try to go too fast or skip steps, you have a greater chance of falling. Habit change is not a race—relax and change a step at a time.

Pause and Consider What Has Been Covered

- Do you have any questions about the Food Diary?
  Yes ______ No ______
  1. The basic task, instructions, reasons for filling it out, how it works, etc? (page 11)
  2. The mechanics of filling it out or questions about definitions? (page 12)

- Did you notice any effect of the Food Diary on your eating?
  Yes ______ No ______ Perhaps

- Be sure to fill out the diary after each meal. Some people carry a pocket notebook, others a 3 X 5 card in their pocket, while others tear out and fold up the diary pages and carry them around. The immediacy of filling it out, and considering what you have eaten after each meal, is very important. If the papers get greasy or have tomato soup on them, that's O.K.—they're for your use—use them in whatever way helps you.

- From now on, do not include coffee, tea, or diet drinks, if they have no calories and do not lead to further eating. (The first week you kept track of *all* eating behaviors so you could establish your eating baseline.)

- If you miss a day, that is O.K. Start again the next meal. Filling it out will become more natural with time. Being aware of the food you are eating is one of the strongest of all habits you can develop to limit your food intake. It is possible to extend the concept of a food diary ahead in time and use it to plan in advance for snacks and meals. The method for doing this will be presented in a later lesson.

- The food diary will change from week to week depending on the topic at hand. I have eliminated some of the columns in the diary for this week, in order to focus your attention on what I feel to be the vital part of today's lesson.

NEW TOPIC: HOME DECALORIZATION—ENVIRONMENTAL CONTROL

Home is where it's at! Home is where we store food, think about food, prepare food, and eat food. This is the environment in which we snack, hide food, cheat, and fool ourselves and others into thinking we are on a diet. This is the environment over which we can have the most control. This is our *own* environment. We want to make it as low-calorie and fat-free as possible, and supportive of our weight loss program.

Last week you took the first step toward eliminating excess food from home. You drew a blueprint of your house, and marked it like a treasure map—except that the X's showed stored food, not buried treasure. (Many would argue that hidden chocolates are a treasure—but not for this program.) A lot of the X's were probably next to the "S" and "M" marks. It is not coincidental that the X's, S's, and M's often occur together. You tend to eat where you find food.

- How many X's are outside the kitchen? ____________
- If you asked for help locating the food, who in the family was the most effective in finding these "mother lodes" of food and extra eating around the house? ____________
- Were you surprised at how widespread your eating was? Yes ______ No ______
- Did you remember those gum drops (25 calories each), that lemonade (150 calories) and that handfull of dry roasted peanuts (200 calories) consumed in front of the TV, while you paused—standing to watch "just for a second"?

This program does not focus on increasing will power and trying to resist food, but on rearranging the environment, and in this way producing changes in your own behavior. For example, if you always respond to the sight of pretzels by first going on a binge of eating the pretzels and then progressing to other snacks, and then being down on yourself for lack of self control, it doesn't make any sense to fight with "will power." The more direct (and more effective) way is to remove the pretzels. If you never see pretzels, you will lose the habit, and they will lose their extra strong appeal.

Research has shown that overweight people are more sensitive to many aspects of their environment than their thin counterparts. (2) This increased sensitivity is a mixed blessing. People who are overweight are more likely to respond to external cues, such as the sight or smell of food, a television ad, the time of day, or a certain place at home which has been associated with food—by eating. At the same time they are less likely to respond to internal cues for eating, like hunger.

Working to change the external world pays off—it removes many of these cues, and teaches you ways of dealing with some of them you cannot change, like time of day, or social situations.

Do You See How This Applies to You?

- Have you ever thought you might be more sensitive to stimuli for cues to eat than the people around you? Yes ______ No ______
- Do you eat when you are not hungry? Yes ______ No ______
- What are some of the things or cues that start you eating?

  1. ______
  2. ______
  3. ______

- Do you see how learning a new set of behaviors and rearranging the world around you a little bit can help you avoid some of those cues or reminders to eat?
  Yes ______ No ______

HOMEWORK

This week we will work on removing the stimulus of food itself, and we want everyone in on the act. Go around the house to all of those X's and move the food to an appropriate storage place. Take the candy from on top of the television and put it in a cupboard in the kitchen. Take the peanuts from beside the bed and put them in the pantry. Go through the house with a finetooth comb to collect all of the food and return it to where it belongs.

Before you put it away, though, consider whether you want to keep it. Does George really need his pretzels within reach, or even within the house for the next few months? Does Johnny have to have his Twinkies when he comes home from school, or could he do just as well with some carrots, or even low-calorie sorbet? And how about those chocolates hidden in your closet? And the cookies on hand just in case the neighbors drop by?

Review your priorities, and look at the junk food you've collected. George will survive, Johnny will get by in school, and the neighbors will probably still love you even if you don't feed them. Make a decision either to store the food out of sight, or throw it away. Decalorize your whole environment, make it safe, and win the war on fat.

Make sure there are no reminders. Remember the sight of food, and the smell of food are problem cues or signals that turn on inappropriate appetite. We'll learn more about this in the next lesson. In the meantime, remember the old saying: "When it's out of sight, it's out of mind."

This week I have simplified the food diary to concentrate on hunger sensations you experience while you are eating. Fill it out as you did last week, with the time, and minutes spent eating, whether it was a meal or a snack, and how hungry you were when you ate it.

Use last week's blueprint of the house to help you prepare a calorie-free environment. Take a red pen, or highliter, and mark each location that you "fat proofed"—from which you removed food.

The homework assignment for this week is:

A. Remove all food from inappropriate storage places throughout the house.

B. Complete the Lesson Two Food Diary.

C. If any new insights or observations come to mind, write them in the column labeled "Comments."

FOOD DIARY — Lesson Two

Sample

Day of Week Monday Date ____________

Time	Minutes Spent Eating	Meal/ Snack	Degree of Hunger	Comments
6:00				
7:20–7:30	10 min	M	2	
8:15–8:20	5 min	S	1	Donut at work
10:30–?	5 min.	S	1	Coffee Break
11:00				
12:30	1 min	S	0	I didn't need this
3:30–3:40	10 min	M	3	Hamburger on the run
4:00				
5:30–6	½ hr	S	2	Restless
6–7	1 hr.	M	1	Little appetite for dinner
9:00				
10:30–10:45	15 min	S	2	Thought I needed for sleep

Degree of Hunger (0 = None, 1 = Some, 2 = Normal, 3 = Good Healthy Hunger, 4 = Ravenous)

FOOD DIARY — Lesson Two

Day of Week ______________________ Date ______________________

Time	Minutes Spent Eating	Meal/ Snack	Degree of Hunger	Comments
6:00				
11:00				
4:00				
9:00				

Degree of Hunger (0 = None, 1 = Some, 2 = Normal, 3 = Good Healthy Hunger, 4 = Ravenous)

FOOD DIARY — Lesson Two

Day of Week ____________________ Date ____________________

Time	Minutes Spent Eating	Meal/ Snack	Degree of Hunger	Comments
6:00				
11:00				
4:00				
9:00				

Degree of Hunger (0 = None, 1 = Some, 2 = Normal, 3 = Good Healthy Hunger, 4 = Ravenous)

FOOD DIARY — Lesson Two

Day of Week ______________________ Date ______________________

Time	Minutes Spent Eating	Meal/ Snack	Degree of Hunger	Comments
6:00				
11:00				
4:00				
9:00				

Degree of Hunger (0 = None, 1 = Some, 2 = Normal, 3 = Good Healthy Hunger, 4 = Ravenous)

FOOD DIARY — Lesson Two

Day of Week ______________________ Date ______________________

Time	Minutes Spent Eating	Meal/ Snack	Degree of Hunger	Comments
6:00				
11:00				
4:00				
9:00				

Degree of Hunger (0 = None, 1 = Some, 2 = Normal, 3 = Good Healthy Hunger, 4 = Ravenous)

FOOD DIARY — Lesson Two

Day of Week ________________ Date ________________

Time	Minutes Spent Eating	Meal/ Snack	Degree of Hunger	Comments
6:00				
11:00				
4:00				
9:00				

Degree of Hunger (0 = None, 1 = Some, 2 = Normal, 3 = Good Healthy Hunger, 4 = Ravenous)

FOOD DIARY — Lesson Two

Day of Week ______________________ Date ______________________

Time	Minutes Spent Eating	Meal/ Snack	Degree of Hunger	Comments
6:00				
11:00				
4:00				
9:00				

Degree of Hunger (0 = None, 1 = Some, 2 = Normal, 3 = Good Healthy Hunger, 4 = Ravenous)

FOOD DIARY — Lesson Two

Day of Week ____________________ Date ____________________

Time	Minutes Spent Eating	Meal/ Snack	Degree of Hunger	Comments
6:00				
11:00				
4:00				
9:00				

Degree of Hunger (0 = None, 1 = Some, 2 = Normal, 3 = Good Healthy Hunger, 4 = Ravenous)

LESSON THREE

CUE ELIMINATION— THE SIGNALS THAT LEAD YOU ASTRAY

WEIGH-IN AND HOMEWORK

Weigh yourself and record your weight on the Personal Weight Record like you did last week. Subtract today's weight from last week's weight, and also from your original baseline weight, and place the figures in the boxes labeled weight change, and total weight change, respectively. Put a dot on the weight loss graph to mark today's weight, and connect it with last week's dot to chart any weight change.

With self-monitoring, you will find that you become much more aware of your eating habits, and possibly more reluctant to eat when you are not actually hungry. In the homework for Lesson One, you kept track of eating episodes, where you ate, and a variety of other measures. You may have found that by simply jotting this information down in a diary, that you lost weight. Many research studies have shown this to average 1/2 to 1-1/2 lbs. the first week (with a slower loss during subsequent weeks). It is a technique that works through increased awareness.

- Did you become more aware of your habits?
  Yes________ No________

- Did you become more aware of places in the environment or individuals around you that seem to trigger eating episodes?
  Yes________ No________

- Did you find yourself eating when you weren't hungry?
  Yes_______ No_______

During the second week you "decalorized" your home environment. You used your home "blueprint," and enlisted the aid of all your family members to hunt down and round up all extra food in the house. Perhaps it's unfair to say "extra," because you were asked to make a judgment about each item and its possible trade-off—whether or not the pretzels really would keep George from straying from home, keep the neighbors from moving out of the neighborhood (or from defacing your property), and keep Johnny from having a temper tantrum after school. At any event, the food that you felt to be necessary was to be stored out of sight in the kitchen—the rest thrown away.

- Did you have difficulty doing this? Yes_______ No_______

- Was it difficult to enlist the aid of family members in this exercise? Yes_______ No_______

- Guess the total number of calories that were removed from around the house and taken into the kitchen:_______calories

- Approximately what percentage of these calories were thrown away?_______%

- Did you get your family to agree not to replace these foods for the duration of your weight loss program?
  Yes_______ No_______

Over the years food creeps into all of our environments. You're working late at night, so a few pieces of candy go into the desk drawer. You're feeling a bit lonely, so that half a box of chocolates got hidden in the closet. You're tired after school, so the extra Twinkie gets stuck away in the bedroom just in case we should have a "hypoglycemic attack."

This type of behavior is very common. Unfortunately it leads to easy accessability of food. Usually this hidden food is calorically dense—after all, who ever bothered to hide a carrot or a stalk of celery in their desk drawer? When the impulse to eat comes, there it is. You're helpless. By moving it to the kitchen, however, and getting rid of as much of it as possible, you can cut down on the extra calories eaten by impulse.

You also kept a food diary last week.

- How many episodes of eating occurred at a hunger level of below 3? ______

- How many episodes of eating occurred at a hunger level between 1 and 0? ______

In our society it's rare for anybody to wait until their hunger level is at 3 or 4. We live in a world of plentiful food and easy accessability. Most habitual eating is unrelated to hunger. It is more related to the environment—the presence or reminders of food—or to an emotional state.

- Add up all the hunger ratings for last week, and find their average. Average hunger for the week ______

- Do the same for week one. Average hunger for week one ______

- What was your average degree of hunger for your snacks for week one______and week two______?

- How many times did you get really hungry (and feel like a member of the Donner Party stranded in the mountains with nothing to eat for a month)?______

If you would only eat when your hunger was at level 3, you would rapidly lose weight. By reducing the impulse eating, you will work toward hungry eating. It's too much to ask this to happen by tomorrow, though. We are creatures of habit. To break these habits takes time and a lot of hard work. That's what this book is all about.

NEW TOPIC: CUE ELIMINATION—GETTING RID OF THOSE RED FLAGS THAT SIGNAL "TIME TO EAT"

Most of our eating is controlled by our psychology, rather than a physical hunger. We have all had the experience of walking down the street after a completely ample breakfast, thinking nothing of food until we walked past a bakery and became aware of the odor of freshly baked bread. At that point all the juices turn on, and the "hunger mechanism," or at least that part of our brain that says "I want some," starts screaming. We at least have to go in to see what smells so good—then ... "oh well."

This is an example of an external cue, something in the environment that stimulates our desire for food. As creatures of habit, over the years we have built up many associations between our eating and the world. Some of these include the time of day, which we dignify with words like breakfast-*time* and dinner-*time*, a variety of places in the house, television shows, advertisements, and the sight and smell of food itself.

One of the most common, but least thought about cues to continue eating beyond one's needs, is the sight of food remaining on the table. It is almost as though there is a need to finish the food in front of us, perhaps as a result of childhood training, or a feeling of guilt, or desire to hoard, or a fear that it won't be there tomorrow.

Food advertisements are excellent examples of external stimuli that try to get us to eat, when we are not hungry, and foods that we might not otherwise want. For the dieter, it's an unfair battle. Food companies spend millions of dollars to find ways to tickle our imagination and turn on our hunger. The dieter is usually passive in this process, and falls into the psychological trap, which is often tastily baited with a food product that may lead one more stretch down the road to obesity.

We also respond to internal cues for eating. Many of us have learned to associate feeling states with eating. Students for example often will munch on crackers, or other foods when studying for exams. There are as many explanations and rationalizations for this as there are students, the most common being "it makes me relax," "makes me think better," "gives me energy," "clears my mind," "keeps me awake," "helps me remember," "gives me extra energy," or "helps me fall asleep." A little self-examination reveals how all of us respond to our internal and external environments by eating unnecessary, extra food.

In the second lesson you learned that overweight people are more sensitive, and seem to be under a greater degree of situational or stimulus control than non-overweight people. That is, you are more likely than a thin friend to feel hungry when you see or smell food—you are more sensitive to these stimuli.

But this sensitivity is not limited to stimuli directly related to foods. The environmental cues that stimulate the sensation of hunger can include the time of day, the television set, the telephone, or your car. Any neutral stimulus in the environment, if paired for a long enough time with eating, can begin to cause the sensation of hunger.

You may have heard of Pavlov's dogs. These animals learned to salivate at the sound of a bell. They did this because they learned to expect food when they heard the experimenter ring his bell. Part of their anticipation of food was salivation. You might say, the sound of the bell made them hungry.

Humans have the same type of reaction to events connected with food. One patient realized, after looking at her food diary, that she always felt hungry when she came in the front door of her house. For years she had followed entering the house with a trip to the refrigerator and snacking. She had paired entering the front door with eating for so long that the front door had become a stimulus for hunger.

Her hunger, of course, had nothing to do with how physically hungry her body was or how low her blood sugar might have been. It was aroused solely by entering the house through the front door. She never experienced this hunger when she came in the back door.

Time itself can become the cue to eat. The sensitivity of overweight people to time was shown very vividly in a series of ingenious psychology experiments by Leonard Schacter. (3) He wanted to see if there was any difference between the perceived passage of time and hunger. His basic tool was a pair of peculiar clocks, one of which ran at half normal speed, the other at twice normal speed. The experiments were carried out at 5:00 in the evening, and were presented to the subjects as studies of their personalities and nervous systems.

After removing each subject's watch, and attaching wires that went to a machine which supposedly measured nervous activity, they left the subject alone in the room with one of the special clocks on the wall.

In one of the two rooms, the experimenter came back into the room when the slow clock read 5:20; in the other, he came back when the fast clock read 6:05. In each case the real time elapsed was 30 minutes. When the experimenter entered the room, he was nibbling on crackers from a box. He set the box down in front of the subject, invited the subject to help himself, and after removing the wires, gave him a personality test (to reinforce the illusion that he was there for a psycholgical testing). The subject was left alone to take the test and asked simply to drop it off at the office on his way out of the building.

There were two groups of subjects, one normal weight, the other overweight. What was actually measured was the weight of crackers consumed.

Overweight subjects ate almost twice as much when they thought the time was 6:05 as they did when they thought that it was 5:20. Thin subjects ate fewer crackers at "6:05," because (they later said) they did not want to spoil their dinners.

The study showed that environmental time cues affected the eating of both normal and overweight subjects, but in different ways:

the belief that dinner time had come stimulated snack eating on the part of the overweight subjects, while it inhibited eating in the thin subjects. The real time of day did not seem to matter. Hunger was controlled by what time the subjects believed it was.

These examples, and this one experiment in particular, show the strong effect environmental cues can have on your life, especially on your eating behaviors.

Try to Apply These Ideas to Yourself

- Were you aware of how cues signal people to eat or feel hungry?
  Yes ______ No ______

- Try to think of an example of an environmental cue in your life that provokes hunger—some signal that reminds you to eat or snack. These can be at home, at work, while traveling, studying—at any time or place or connected with any activity.
  List three: 1.______________________________
  2.______________________________
  3.______________________________

(You might be able to identify more of these if you look back at your food diary.)

CUE ELIMINATION—HOW TO DO IT!

The principle behind stimulus control is quite simple. If something turns your sense of hunger on, and that hunger has nothing to do with a bodily state of starvation or hypoglycemia, then learning to ignore that stimulus will eventually return the stimulus to neutral. If the nonresponse is practiced long enough, the stimulus or cue will lose its ability to make you want to eat.

The techniques of cue elimination will require some cooperation from the people around you, both at home and at work. Cue related behaviors are difficult to change, because they often involve other people, especially at home, and may require some changes in the physical arrangement of your household.

At the end of the first lesson you drew a rough plan of your house and indicated on it where each eating episode took place. Most people find clusters of snacks around the television set, by favorite chairs, or in the kitchen by the refrigerator or sink. Last week, you removed food from inappropriate storage places—and either threw it away or put it out of sight in the kitchen or pantry.

How About You?

- Have you noticed any patterns to your eating?
  Yes ________ No ________

- Were there more separate eating places than you anticipated?
  Yes________ No________

Because you are likely to eat in response to external cues, it makes sense that eliminating the cues will break up your eating habits. Thus, if you break the association between TV and eating, watching TV will no longer make you hungry. Similarly, if you do all of your eating in one place in your house, after a while the other places will no longer remind you to eat.

HOMEWORK

Eliminating all of the stimuli which evoke feelings of hunger is difficult, if not impossible in one step. The easiest way to start is with a set of exercises designed to help you eliminate eating cues; they make up a six-part assignment as follows:

1. Choose a specific place in one room of your home to do all of your eating. This will be your *Designated Appropriate Eating Place.* It can be in the kitchen, dining room, or den, and may be different for each meal. It should be a place where you can sit down and eat in relative comfort. From today on, eat all of your meals and snacks at your *Designated Appropriate Eating Place* for each particular meal. When you have meals away from home, such as at work, or when out for a meal, the *Designated Appropriate Eating Place* will be just that—a location that you consider to be an appropriate eating place. This might be a table in a restaurant, cafeteria, or lunchroom.

   Write down your *Designated Appropriate Eating Place.* By writing it down, you are committing yourself to eat in this location. If you don't commit yourself, the chances are you won't change as rapidly. Think about where it will be appropriate (and safe) for you to eat for the next few months, and commit yourself to it now.

- My Designated Appropriate Eating Place for breakfast is:

  ____

- My Designated Appropriate Eating Place for lunch is:

  at home ______________________________

  at work ______________________________

- My Designated Appropriate Eating Place for dinner is:

  ____

- My Designated Appropriate Eating Place for snacks at home is:

  ____

- Other places where I feel it is appropriate to eat, where there will be few inappropriate eating cues:

  ____

  ____

  (for example, a restaurant)

When you eat at work, try to avoid eating at your desk. The object of cue elimination tasks is to break up the association between eating and other activities such as working. If there is no place to eat other than at your desk, at least change it by adding a place mat and silverware and a real cup for your coffee.

Try to make it look different from the place where you work. In one experimental situation researchers discovered that a brightly colored place mat helped people designate an eating place which later became a cue for appropriate eating behaviors. For some people a change of this type at work or home is a great help.

Make your eating place special. From today on eating should be a point of luxury in your life, something to enjoy. Do everything you can to make your eating place pleasant. You can include flowers, music, a comfortable seat, pretty plates, your best silverware—but most important, include enough time. All of these pleasant additions to your eating place will be cues for a new eating style.

2. If your Designated Appropriate Eating Place is the regular dining table, change your habitual eating place at the table. If

you regularly sit at the head of the table, change to the side; if you sit on one side, change places with someone on the other side. This may make things a little less efficient for a while, but it also will break up a lot of longstanding cues at the table. This change need not be forever; just to try for a few weeks and see what happens.

3. When eating, only eat. Don't talk on the phone, watch television, read, work, etc. Concentrate on your food and those with you. I want you to really taste your food, feel the textures, and try to enjoy each mouthful—make each meal enjoyable.

4. Continue to remove food from all places in the house other than appropriate storage areas such as the kitchen. Examples are candy on the television set and nuts in the living room. Don't let it creep back to those "off limits" areas.

   Keep stored food out of sight. This can be done by putting food in cupboards, or keeping it in opaque containers that you cannot see through. Do the same for foods in the refrigerator—put everything in "see-proof" containers. To further reduce the strength of the visual cues, you can put lower wattage bulbs in the kitchen area where you prepare and store food, and replace your refrigerator light with a dim one—or remove it altogether.

5. Have other foods on hand to replace junk or convenience foods—if you must have both in the house, keep one, the healthy one, visible in an attractive container, the empty-calorie food out of sight in a dark container. It will help you decide which to eat when the impulse to snack comes along.

6. Do not keep serving containers on the table while you eat. If this is not possible, put the serving dishes at the other end of the table from where you sit.

The behavior changes introduced in this lesson seem simple—but in practice they are very difficult to master. Eating in one place is awkward at first for many people. Remember to eat only in a place that you designate as appropriate. The object of this exercise is to eliminate cues that you have traditionally associated with food; with time and lack of use these cues will return to a neutral state where food is concerned. Your new eating place will take over this cueing function and it will begin to remind you of a new set of eating behaviors.

FIGURE 2
EATING PLACE RECORD

(Numbers under the days of the week refer to consecutive eating epi

Sample

PLACE	Monday						Tuesday						Wednesday						Thursday						Friday						Saturday						Su		
	1	2	3	4	5	6	1	2	3	4	5	6	1	2	3	4	5	6	1	2	3	4	5	6	1	2	3	4	5	6	1	2	3	4	5	6	1	2	3
Car	■						■									■																							
Office desk		■						■						■						■																			
Den–TV room				■																															■	■			
Living room																						■					■												
Designated eating place			■			■			■	■			■		■			■	■					■	■	■		■					■	■					■
Bedroom											■																		■								■		
Kitchen (not at table)																	■														■								
Other																																■						■	

WEEK 1

PLACE	Monday						Tuesday						Wednesday						Thursday						Friday						Saturday						Su		
	1	2	3	4	5	6	1	2	3	4	5	6	1	2	3	4	5	6	1	2	3	4	5	6	1	2	3	4	5	6	1	2	3	4	5	6	1	2	3
Car																																							
Office desk																																							
Den–TV room																																							
Living room																																							
Designated eating place																																							
Bedroom																																							
Kitchen (not at table)																																							
Other																																							

Make a graph of your week one eating place locations. For the "Designated Eating Place", use the locations you chose earlier this chapter.

You probably will not be able to accomplish these cue elimination exercises immediately, even though they sound very simple. They are not simple for everyone. If you are not completely successful the first week, do not feel guilty or give up. Try to do a little better each day.

Eating Place Record

One way to improve your chances of success is to provide yourself with some form of information about your progress. To help you keep track of your eating locations, I have included a type of graph, a scatter diagram entitled "Eating Place Record." (Figure 2) On it you will find six common eating places listed under "Place," and one additional line labeled "Other," for places not on the list.

Turn back to your Week One Food Diary. Find the column labeled "Location of Eating." Transfer this information for each day of the week to the eating place record. The six numbered columns under each day of the week are for consecutive eating episodes—snacks or meals.

As part of the homework forms for this week you will find an Eating Place Record similar to the one in Figure 2.

Remember, the Designated Appropriate Eating Place will be the place that you have chosen for your meals and snacks. Almost always it will include a table and chair, and it usually will be the same place at least for the same meal each day; for example, the kitchen table for breakfast, a table at the cafeteria at work for lunch, and at the dining room table for dinner. You can include restaurants, lunch rooms, picnics—any place that you feel is appropriate for meals away from home. If you have a snack, take it to the place you have designated as appropriate before you eat it.

Each day, check the box that indicates where each eating episode took place. You can either do this when you eat or when you review your food diary. The ideal is a straight line with the "Designated Appropriate Eating Place" checked for every meal or snack. The closer you can come to this ideal (as shown in the "ideal completed sample"), the closer you will come to eliminating a large number of environmental cues that may be reminding you to eat, or may be making you momentarily hungry when you really aren't.

You will be most sucessful with cue elimination if you have help from your family and friends. Tell them what you are doing and the reasons for it. You will find that explaining the techniques to others will help you understand them better yourself. Your family's enthusiasm can only help.

Many other cues can be eliminated from your immediate environment—all of the little signals that say "*eat*": leftovers, snacks, vending machines, and shopping center treats. A technique can be devised for each of these to eliminate specific causes of impulse eating, and they will be discussed later. This week, however, concentrate on the six exercises introduced earlier.

Food Diary

The final column on the food diary for this lesson is labeled, "Food Out of Sight." Put a "yes" in this column if food was in containers and out of sight before each meal or snack, and if serving containers were not prominent on the table during meals. (If they cannot be taken off the table, arrange for them to be as far away from you as possible—to reduce their effectiveness as a cue.)

In summary, this week you start eliminating cues from your environment that might be triggers for hungry feelings. Food should assume a low profile in your home. The keys to this are: eating in one place; changing your eating place at the table; only eating at mealtimes; removing food from storage areas; having foods on hand to replace junk foods; and removing serving dishes from the table.

The homework assignment for this week is:

A. Lesson Three Food Diary. Mark the last column of the Food Diary "yes" or "no" to indicate whether visual cues were reduced for each meal or snack. Remember, if you are going to eat, make it worthwhile.

B. Designate an appropriate eating place at home and work. Eat all of your meals and snacks at this place.

C. Change your habitual eating place at the table.

D. When eating, only eat. No other activities.

E. Remove food from all places in the house which are not appropriate storage areas. Reduce visual cues for eating. Store food in opaque containers.

F. Keep junk foods out of sight, hidden, hard to get, or don't buy them.

G. Remove serving dishes from the table or put them at the opposite end of the table.

H. Fill in the Eating Place Record for each meal and snack during the past week, and for the next two weeks.

FOOD DIARY — Lesson Three

Sample

Day of Week Monday Date ______________

Time	Minutes Spent Eating	M/S	H	Activity While Eating	Location of Eating	Food Out of Sight yes/no
6:00 7:20 – 7:30	10min	M	0	Paper	Kitchen	Yes
8:15 – 8:20	5min	S	0	Talking	Work	
11:00 3:30 – 3:40	10min	M	3	Reading	Restaurant	Yes
4:00 6-7	1 hr	M	2	T.V	Dining Room	Yes
9:00 10:30– 10:45	15min	3	0	TV	Living Room	Yes

M/S: Meal or Snack; H: Degree of Hunger (0 = None, 1 = Some, 2 = Normal, 3 = Good Healthy Hunger, 4 = Ravenous)

FOOD DIARY — Lesson Three

Day of Week ______________________ Date ______________________

Time	Minutes Spent Eating	M/S	H	Activity While Eating	Location of Eating	Food Out of Sight yes/no
6:00						
11:00						
4:00						
9:00						

M/S: Meal or Snack; H: Degree of Hunger (0 = None, 1 = Some, 2 = Normal, 3 = Good Healthy Hunger, 4 = Ravenous)

FOOD DIARY — Lesson Three

Day of Week ______________ Date ______________

Time	Minutes Spent Eating	M/S	H	Activity While Eating	Location of Eating	Food Out of Sight yes/no
6:00						
11:00						
4:00						
9:00						

M/S: Meal or Snack; H: Degree of Hunger (0 = None, 1 = Some, 2 = Normal, 3 = Good Healthy Hunger, 4 = Ravenous)

FOOD DIARY — Lesson Three

Day of Week ______________ Date ______________

Time	Minutes Spent Eating	M/S	H	Activity While Eating	Location of Eating	Food Out of Sight yes/no
6:00						
11:00						
4:00						
9:00						

M/S: Meal or Snack; H: Degree of Hunger (0 = None, 1 = Some, 2 = Normal, 3 = Good Healthy Hunger, 4 = Ravenous)

FOOD DIARY — Lesson Three

Day of Week ________________ Date ________________

Time	Minutes Spent Eating	M/S	H	Activity While Eating	Location of Eating	Food Out of Sight yes/no
6:00						
11:00						
4:00						
9:00						

M/S: Meal or Snack; H: Degree of Hunger (0 = None, 1 = Some, 2 = Normal, 3 = Good Healthy Hunger, 4 = Ravenous)

FOOD DIARY — Lesson Three

Day of Week ______________________ Date ______________________

Time	Minutes Spent Eating	M/S	H	Activity While Eating	Location of Eating	Food Out of Sight yes/no
6:00						
11:00						
4:00						
9:00						

M/S: Meal or Snack; H: Degree of Hunger (0 = None, 1 = Some, 2 = Normal, 3 = Good Healthy Hunger, 4 = Ravenous)

FOOD DIARY — Lesson Three

Day of Week ______________________ Date ______________________

Time	Minutes Spent Eating	M/S	H	Activity While Eating	Location of Eating	Food Out of Sight yes/no
6:00						
11:00						
4:00						
9:00						

M/S: Meal or Snack; H: Degree of Hunger (0 = None, 1 = Some, 2 = Normal, 3 = Good Healthy Hunger, 4 = Ravenous)

FOOD DIARY — Lesson Three

Day of Week ______________________ Date ______________________

Time	Minutes Spent Eating	M/S	H	Activity While Eating	Location of Eating	Food Out of Sight yes/no
6:00						
11:00						
4:00						
9:00						

M/S: Meal or Snack; H: Degree of Hunger (0 = None, 1 = Some, 2 = Normal, 3 = Good Healthy Hunger, 4 = Ravenous)

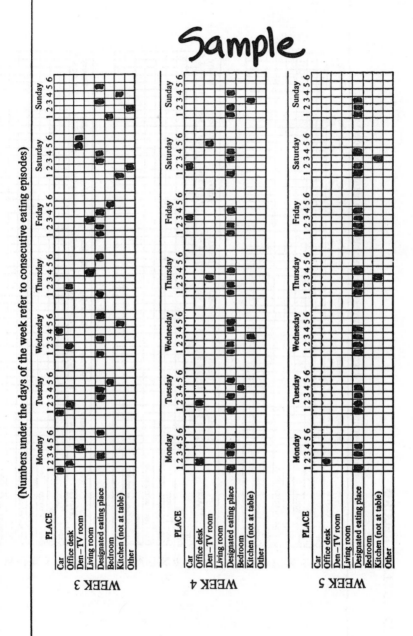

EATING PLACE RECORD

(Numbers under the days of the week refer to consecutive eating episodes)

Sample

WEEK 3

PLACE	Monday 1 2 3 4 5 6	Tuesday 1 2 3 4 5 6	Wednesday 1 2 3 4 5 6	Thursday 1 2 3 4 5 6	Friday 1 2 3 4 5 6	Saturday 1 2 3 4 5 6	Sunday 1 2 3 4 5 6
Car	1	1	4				
Office desk	2	2	2	2			
Den–TV room	4					5, 6	
Living room				4	3		
Designated eating place	3, 6	3, 4	1, 3, 6	1, 6	1, 2, 4	3, 4	3, 5
Bedroom		5			5		1
Kitchen (not at table)			5			1	4
Other						2	2

WEEK 4

PLACE	Monday 1 2 3 4 5 6	Tuesday 1 2 3 4 5 6	Wednesday 1 2 3 4 5 6	Thursday 1 2 3 4 5 6	Friday 1 2 3 4 5 6	Saturday 1 2 3 4 5 6	Sunday 1 2 3 4 5 6
Car					3	2	
Office desk	2	2					
Den–TV room				3		5	
Living room							
Designated eating place	1, 3, 4	1, 3, 5	1, 2, 4, 5	1, 2, 4	1, 2, 4	1, 3, 4	1, 2, 4
Bedroom		4					
Kitchen (not at table)			3				3
Other							

WEEK 5

PLACE	Monday 1 2 3 4 5 6	Tuesday 1 2 3 4 5 6	Wednesday 1 2 3 4 5 6	Thursday 1 2 3 4 5 6	Friday 1 2 3 4 5 6	Saturday 1 2 3 4 5 6	Sunday 1 2 3 4 5 6
Car							
Office desk	2						
Den–TV room							
Living room							
Designated eating place	1, 3, 4	1, 2, 3, 4	1, 2, 3, 4	1, 2, 4	1, 2, 3, 4	1, 2, 4	1, 2, 3
Bedroom							
Kitchen (not at table)				3		3	
Other							

EATING PLACE RECORD

(Numbers under the days of the week refer to consecutive eating episodes)

WEEK 3

PLACE	Monday						Tuesday						Wednesday						Thursday						Friday						Saturday						Sunday					
	1	2	3	4	5	6	1	2	3	4	5	6	1	2	3	4	5	6	1	2	3	4	5	6	1	2	3	4	5	6	1	2	3	4	5	6	1	2	3	4	5	6
Car																																										
Office desk																																										
Den–TV room																																										
Living room																																										
Designated eating place																																										
Bedroom																																										
Kitchen (not at table)																																										
Other																																										

WEEK 4

PLACE	Monday						Tuesday						Wednesday						Thursday						Friday						Saturday						Sunday					
	1	2	3	4	5	6	1	2	3	4	5	6	1	2	3	4	5	6	1	2	3	4	5	6	1	2	3	4	5	6	1	2	3	4	5	6	1	2	3	4	5	6
Car																																										
Office desk																																										
Den–TV room																																										
Living room																																										
Designated eating place																																										
Bedroom																																										
Kitchen (not at table)																																										
Other																																										

WEEK 5

PLACE	Monday						Tuesday						Wednesday						Thursday						Friday						Saturday						Sunday					
	1	2	3	4	5	6	1	2	3	4	5	6	1	2	3	4	5	6	1	2	3	4	5	6	1	2	3	4	5	6	1	2	3	4	5	6	1	2	3	4	5	6
Car																																										
Office desk																																										
Den–TV room																																										
Living room																																										
Designated eating place																																										
Bedroom																																										
Kitchen (not at table)																																										
Other																																										

LESSON FOUR

BEING ACTIVE—THE DIFFERENCE BETWEEN SUCCESS AND FAILURE

WEIGH-IN AND HOMEWORK

Weigh yourself and record your weight. Calculate and plot your weight change on your Personal Weight Record. (The average weight change at this point in the program is roughly three pounds. This is shown by the solid diagonal line across the graph on your Personal Weight Record.)

Check your homework for Lesson Three and record whether or not you completed it on the Homework Credit Sheet.

- Is your Lesson Three Food Diary complete?
  Yes_______ No_______
- Is the "Food Out of Sight" column in the Food Diary checked for every day? Yes_______ No_______
- Is your Eating Place Record filled in for this week?
  Yes_______ No_______

REVIEW

This program stresses eating behaviors rather than nutrition or calories. Although there has been no discussion of *self-observation* as such, it has been your prime method of assessing eating behaviors. You have kept meticulous track of your food intake, the time, place, and reasons for eating, in addition to records of the type of food you eat. This recording has sensitized you to your eating behaviors and has made you very aware of your eating patterns.

The food diary has been the principal tool in helping you change your perception of food. It can be a very powerful aid in reshaping your eating habits and maintaining these habits once they have been established.

How Are You Doing?

- Are you keeping track of your food intake on the food diary forms? Yes______ No______

- Are you having difficulty filling out the diary? Yes______ No______ (See page 12)

- Are you giving yourself credit for completed homework? Yes______ No______

- Many people can see emerging patterns of eating behaviors, and changes in their eating habits by this point in the program—can you? Yes______ No______

- During the second lesson you removed excess calories from the world around you—and you began to exert control over your environment. If you made a check now, would there be any food in:

  a. the TV room? Yes______ No______
  b. the family room? Yes______ No______
  c. the bedroom? Yes______ No______
  d. the car? Yes______ No______

During the third lesson you learned that overweight people are more sensitive than thin people to environmental stimuli, to those little reminders around you that signal "Eat." These cues include places, times, events, emotions, and social situations. Any object, feeling or place can become a reminder to eat, and can evoke hunger if it is paired with food for a long enough period of time. Some examples given were television programs, the refrigerator, and, in one case, the front door.

The cue-elimination part of the homework assignment for this past week had six parts, each designed to disconnect a set of cue-related eating patterns. These were:

1. Choosing a Designated Appropriate Eating Place.
2. Switching places at the table.
3. Doing nothing else when eating.
4. Making food less visible by storing it in opaque containers, and removing food from other areas in the house.
5. Minimizing the attraction of "junk," or "empty-calorie" foods.
6. Taking serving dishes off the table.

Choosing the Designated Appropriate Eating Place was emphasized particularly, because it is often the most useful in breaking habits. We provided you with an Eating Place Record or scatter diagram, to keep track of where your meals and snacks were eaten. It is a tool to help you change. A straight line across from your Designated Appropriate Eating Place indicates you were at your designated place every time you had something to eat.

How Do You Feel About That Assignment?

- Was there any difficulty continuing with the assignment the second week? Yes_______ No_______
- Do you understand what this homework assignment was supposed to accomplish? Yes_______ No_______
- Is it becoming easier to eat in only one place? Yes_______ No_______

It is important to practice all of the cue elimination exercises every time you have something to eat. Check the following to see how well you are doing:

	Yes	No
A. Are you storing food in opaque containers?	______	______
B. Did you acquire special "see-proof" containers for food?	______	______

C. Is food more out of sight at home now than before? ____ ____

D. Is junk food either not purchased or kept out of sight? ____ ____

E. Are you doing nothing else when you eat? ____ ____

F. What are some of your remaining cues for eating, and what can be done to eliminate them?

1. ____________________

2. ____________________

In the coming months, you will find the strength of old environmental cues diminishing. Many people report that 12 to 15 weeks of cue elimination practice are necessary to return strong cues, like television, to neutral. At that point the cue no longer makes them hungry and does not remind them of food.

The Theory of Behavior Modification

Last week's lesson reviewed the theory of behavior modification and the concept of over-eating as a learned behavior. Since eating behaviors are learned, the logical way to change them is to learn competing or opposing behaviors, or to change the environment in a way which will eliminate the associated behavior. The effect on the original habits is that without practice they become weaker, and eventually are weakened or extinguished.

It is very important to *be consistent*. If you practice not eating in front of the television set for three weeks, and then start again, you will very rapidly reestablish your old association of television with food, and television may re-emerge as an even stronger environmental cue than before.

Eliminating Environmental Cues

Last week much of the discussion concerned the effect of environmental cues on eating behaviors. Many kinds of cues were identified: place cues, activity cues, time cues, and emotional cues. Any stimulus (place, event, or feeling) paired long enough with eating will signal you to feel hunger, or to want to eat when you encounter it. The technique of cue elimination was introduced as a systematic way of breaking up these patterns of cue and response. If you no longer eat after you open the refrigerator, the refrigerator will, with time, lose the hunger-provoking quality it may have now.

You drew a house plan and marked on it every place where you had either a meal or a snack. The object of this exercise was to give you a graphic representation of where you eat, and to provide a way of analyzing the cues that surround you. Most people find they eat in different places throughout the house, and some are able to see from the house plan which cues are telling them to eat.

Several exercises in cue elimination were introduced, which have been designed to break up the associations between eating cues and eating responses at home:

1. The technique most emphasized last week was choosing a specific place (or if necessary, more than one) for your eating—your *Designated Appropriate Eating Place*—and eating all of your meals and snacks there. For meals eaten out of the house, for example at work, such a place might have to be a restaurant, or some other place you feel is appropriate. This is a behavior change that is difficult, because it is a major change and involves other members of the family.

   You filled in a scatter diagram Eating Place Record to help you with this change. The object of the diagram was to give you immediate feedback about the location of your meals and snacks. You could see how well you were doing by how close you came to recording a straight line on your Eating Place Record.

Let's Consider the Eating Place Record for a Moment.

- Did you understand how to fill it out?
  Yes_______ No_______ (page 53)

- Did you achieve a straight line on the diagram?
  Yes_______ No_______

- Did you notice any effect of this technique on the amount you ate last week? Yes_______ No_______

2. You were asked to *change places with someone at the table* to see how different the meals look from another vantage point. A side effect of this technique is to make you extra aware of mealtime, of the changes that are going on in your eating habits, and to provide the social setting for change. Everyone at the table will be aware of your change, and this can give you a starting point for eating differently.

How Did This Work Out?

- Did you experience any difference changing from your customary eating place? Yes_______ No_______

- Any comment from your family? Yes_______ No_______

- Was it helpful? Yes_______ No_______

- What did you do to make your eating place special?

  1. ______________________________
  2. ______________________________

3. You were to *only eat during mealtimes*, avoiding any associated activity not appropriate to enjoying a good meal. You were to concentrate on your food, to try to be a gourmet, to taste and try to enjoy every mouthful. The reason for this was to break up associations between activities like reading a paper in the mid-morning and hunger. When you are hungry, only eat.

How Did This Go?

- Did you pay more attention to your meals as a result of this technique? Yes_______ No_______

- Do you remember why this is such an important exercise? Yes_______ No_______

It is very important that you continue applying this technique. It becomes easier with time. You will find meals will be more enjoyable, food tastier, and conversation more lively without the television. Doing without diversions is difficult at first, but it gets easier.

4. Next, you were to *remove all food from non-storage places* in the house—for example, by the bed or on top of the television set. The reason for this was to remove the cue of food itself from your home environment. This should have been easy, because you located all of your eating places on your house plan last week.

   In addition to putting food in proper storage areas, you were to make food less visible. Some of the techniques suggested were putting food in opaque containers, putting dim bulbs in food preparation areas, and putting a smaller light in your refrigerator (or taking it out altogether). All of these tactics help you counteract the hunger cues built into the sight of food. When food is stored conspicuously, it looks and smells more appealing and it makes you hungry. When it is out of sight, it no longer has this power. You were asked to keep track in your food diary of attempts to keep food out of sight.

Was There Any Trouble?

- This technique often involves the family, and sometimes it requires their cooperation to get the potato chips out of the family room. Did you encounter any family resistance? Yes______ No______
- Will it be difficult to continue keeping food in the proper storage places? Yes______ No______
- Did you put your food in opaque ("see-proof") containers? Yes______ No______
- Did you go all the way and take the bulb out of your refrigerator? Yes______ No______

5. You were urged to keep low-calorie foods on hand if necessary for the sudden urges to eat. *High-impulse or junk foods* should either not be purchased, or at least be kept in a place where they cannot reach out and grab your appetite—for example, in a dark container or, if appropriate, in the freezer.

- Did you put junk foods out of sight? Yes______ No______
- Did you throw junk food away? Yes______ No______

6. Another technique to decrease impulse eating is to *remove serving dishes from the table*. If this proved impossible, you were to place them at the end of the table farthest away from you, to minimize their effect on your eating.

Was This Helpful?

- Were you able to do this? Yes______ No______
- Did your family object to this? Yes______ No______

If you haven't been able to use all of these techniques in one week, don't worry; it is not a setback. Everyone goes at his or her own pace. More time may be needed to change what for you might be a more difficult or stronger habit than for someone else. If you feel you need it, take another week and work on them, until you feel satisfied that they are mastered—then go on.

Be creative in your solutions. There are many ways to go about cue elimination. When you become aware of eating in response to a cue in your environment, any place or any time, try to disassociate it from eating and food.

I will keep referring to a particular point in connection with *all* of the changes in behaviors you make in this course: the important concept of "Maintenance." If you don't keep track of new behaviors, they fade away with time. If they don't persist, they won't help.

In a few weeks I will introduce a checklist for new behaviors, so you can monitor yourself and insure that your new behaviors are continuing. This mechanical checking can be reduced or eliminated with time, but while the changes are fresh, I will ask you to check your behaviors daily—then eventually to change to weekly or monthly self-evaluation. For the next week though, keep working on the cue elimination assignments and filling in the Eating Place Record, in addition to the weekly food diary.

NEW TOPIC: BEING ACTIVE

"A bear, however hard he tries,
Grows tubby without exercise.
Our Teddy bear is short and fat,
Which is not to be wondered at;
He gets what exercise he can
By falling off the ottoman,
But generally seems to lack
The energy to clamber back.*"

Many of us feel like "Edward Bear"—we sit, grow rounder, and once dislodged, barely have the energy to clamber back to our seat. Exercise is a key ingredient of a weight loss program. Without it, weight loss is often wishful thinking. It is a powerful tool in weight control, and building it into a weight loss program can be the difference between failure and success. Exercise burns calories directly, but it also affects the calories you burn metabolically.

As calories diminish, so does metabolic rate (so your body burns less energy at rest). This makes weight loss slower, as your

***When We Were Very Young*, by A. A. Milne. Copyright 1924 by E.P. Dutton, renewed 1952 by A.A. Milne. Reprinted by permission of the publisher, E.P. Dutton, a division of NAL Penguin Inc.

metabolism becomes more efficient. Your body clings to every calorie more tightly, and if there are extra calories, they are stashed away as fat more readily. Exercise can counteract some of this effect, by raising your metabolic rate.

Fill in the following sentences:

I hate exercise because ______________________________

____

When others see me exercising, they think ________________

____

I don't exercise enough now because ___________________

____

I would be more likely to exercise if ___________________

____

Look at your answers. They may be standing between you and weight loss. Consider them carefully, and whether or not you are willing to give up what they represent, to help burn more calories.

Let's consider excuses. Among the more common reasons people don't exercise are, "I can't compete with others," and "I'm not coordinated"—neither of which is relevant. Exercise is for yourself.

You also may have found yourself saying, "I exercised and hurt myself." This often happens, particularly with the overweight. Take it easy. Start with walking, and build up slowly. You won't run a marathon the first week, but you won't injure yourself either.

Then there is, "I am embarrassed when people see me exercising." You can exercise in private, or you may learn to take pride in the fact that people will be watching as you lose weight, and patting you on the back. If this external motivation feels good, it can help your commitment to an exercise and weight reduction program. The praise of others can be a powerful stimulus to help keep you going.

Finally, there is the universal, "I haven't enough time." It's a matter of priorities, and you may have to make a substitution. For instance, time previously spent looking for snack foods could be devoted to physical activities. A goal of this program will be to help you learn to incorporate many types of physical activity into your daily life.

ENERGY: PART ONE

(You will need a pedometer for this and subsequent lessons. They can be purchased at sporting goods, variety, and fitness specialty stores.)

A simple equation can be written for how to gain and lose weight. It holds true for everyone—and the entire animal kingdom:

ENERGY IN (food) = ENERGY USED (activity*) + STORAGE (fa

Increasing Activity

So far you have worked on the "energy in" side of the equation, by modifying your intake and thus reducing the amount of energy consumed. Up to now, by reducing the amount on the intake side of the equation, you have also reduced the total amount on the other side. Even if your activity hasn't changed, if you've reduced intake energy below activity energy, some of your storage energy (fat) has been burned up. Now, if you can actually increase your activity, even more fat will be burned up.

For the next two weeks you will be working on the other side of the equation—"energy used"—through activity. To understand this topic most meaningfully, you will have to think in terms of calories. However, the calories you are concerned with in this lesson are those used up rather than those eaten.

This week I want to introduce the topic of energy use and have you make some observations about your activity. In the next lesson I will talk more about energy use and introduce some techniques to increase energy expenditure (without calisthenics).

Additions to exercise, either as a planned event or through a general increase in physical activity, can be among the hardest behaviors to build into one's routine. Lying on the couch or sitting in front of television can be very pleasant compared to moving about, expecially if you're overweight and out of shape.

If your only activity is watching television, it may be of some comfort to know that your Basal Metabolic Rate, the amount of energy consumed through basal metabolism while you are resting, increases 20 percent if you sit rather than lie down to watch TV; it increases even more if you stand rather than sit—unfortunately not many people like to stand while they watch TV.

Too many people believe that exercise plays only a minor role in losing weight. After all, even jogging only burns up ten calories per minute. Actually an increased expenditure of energy is very impor-

*Actually, your body burns some energy while completely at rest, because of your basal metabolism—generally all the processes that just keep your body alive and functioning.

tant to weight loss programs. Regular exercise should increase the rate of weight loss throughout a weight loss program, and for many people who have reached a plateau, exercise can reestablish their downward trend.

There is recent evidence that the increased energy expenditure level persists for a period after the actual exercise. But most importantly, regular exercise may change your body "set point" to a lower level by increasing your metabolic ("idling") rate, so that you burn more calories even when at rest. This won't happen after the first time around the track—but when it does, it will help make weight control much easier.

Contrary to popular belief, expending more energy usually does not lead to an increase in appetite. Studies have shown that food intake actually decreases when the average person increases his or her level of physical activity. (5) Because of this, exercise can actually contribute to the ease of food restriction in weight loss programs.

This week you will analyze some of your activities and begin to think about their caloric "worth." Remember that an extra 250 calories burned each day is equal to one-half pound of weight loss a week, or 26 pounds lost each year, with no change in food intake.

HOMEWORK

During the coming week, you will collect two types of data to give yourself a baseline or starting point for next week's lesson:

1. Record (on the Daily Activity Record at the end of this lesson) the number of minutes you spend each day in physical activity *in addition* to the activity of your daily routine. Examples of extra activities would be gardening, golfing, running, swimming, and moving furniture. Next week you will convert these minutes of exercise to their caloric equivalent to help you make some changes that will burn up extra calories. (Do not fill in the spaces marked "Calories." You will do that next lesson.)
2. Keep track of the number of miles you walk each day. Wear your pedometer and record your miles per day on your Daily Activity Record.

The pedometer converts the up and down motion of your body when you walk, to a measure of distance. (Inside the pedometer is a small pendulum that moves up and down with each step you take. These movements of the pendulum are translated by gears into a series of small movements of the needle on the face of the pedometer.

The farther you walk, the more up and down movements, and the more distance registered on the dial.)

To use the pedometer accurately, you must program it for the length of your stride. This allows the device to calculate the distance you have traveled on the basis of your number of steps and the average length of each step. Your stride is determined by counting the number of steps you make in a standard distance, and dividing this into the distance walked. For example, if you take 50 steps when you walk a distance of 100 feet, the length of your stride is two feet (100 feet divided by 50 steps = 2 feet per step).

Set the pedometer for the length of your stride. Every evening write down the number of miles you have walked during the day. After you write down your mileage, turn the meter back to zero to start the next day's recording.

Next week you will calculate your current activity level, and you will be given some strategies to help you increase your daily energy expenditure.

Is This All Clear?

- Do you understand the energy equation and terms used in it? Yes_______ No_______ (page 74)

- Be sure you understand the assignment and how to use the pedometer before you begin this week's assignment. If necessary, ask someone at a sport shop to help you adjust it. Once it is adjusted, don't change it.

The homework assignment for this week is:

A. Complete the Lesson Four Food Diary.

B. Keep your food out of sight.

C. Continue to blacken in the appropriate box on your Eating Place Record (Lesson Three, page 52). Make it form a straight line this week! If eating at your Designated Appropriate Eating Place has only become comfortable for one meal a day, try to increase by a second meal or snack.

D. Write down on the Daily Activity Record the miles you walk each day, as well as the number of minutes spent in non-routine exercise. Do not fill in the space marked "Calories."

FOOD DIARY — Lesson Four

Sample

Day of Week ____________ Date ____________

Daily Activity Record Completed? yes ✓ no ___ Food Out of Sight? yes ✓ no ___

Time	M/S	H	Location of Eating	Comments
6:00				
7:15	m	2	Kitchen	
8:30	S	0	Cafeteria	Sweet Roll & Coffee
11:00				
12:30	M	3	Cafeteria	
4:00				
4:30	S	1	Restaurant	Pick-me-up
7:15	m	2	Dining Room	
9:00				
9:15	S	0	TV Room	lousy TV

M/S: Meal or Snack; H: Degree of Hunger (0 = None, 1 = Some, 2 = Normal, 3 = Good Healthy Hunger, 4 = Ravenous)

FOOD DIARY — Lesson Four

Day of Week ______________________ Date ______________________

Daily Activity Record Completed? yes___ no ___ Food Out of Sight? yes ___no ___

Time	M/S	H	Location of Eating	Comments
6:00				
11:00				
4:00				
9:00				

M/S: Meal or Snack; H: Degree of Hunger (0 = None, 1 = Some, 2 = Normal, 3 = Good Healthy Hunger, 4 = Ravenous)

FOOD DIARY — Lesson Four

Day of Week ____________________ Date ____________________

Daily Activity Record Completed? yes___ no ___ Food Out of Sight? yes ___no ___

Time	M/S	H	Location of Eating	Comments
6:00				
11:00				
4:00				
9:00				

M/S: Meal or Snack; H: Degree of Hunger (0 = None, 1 = Some, 2 = Normal, 3 = Good Healthy Hunger, 4 = Ravenous)

FOOD DIARY — Lesson Four

Day of Week ______________________ Date ______________________

Daily Activity Record Completed? yes___ no ___ Food Out of Sight? yes ___no ___

Time	M/S	H	Location of Eating	Comments
6:00				
11:00				
4:00				
9:00				

M/S: Meal or Snack; H: Degree of Hunger (0 = None, 1 = Some, 2 = Normal, 3 = Good Healthy Hunger, 4 = Ravenous)

FOOD DIARY — Lesson Four

Day of Week ____________________ Date ____________________

Daily Activity Record Completed? yes___ no___ Food Out of Sight? yes ___no ___

Time	M/S	H	Location of Eating	Comments
6:00				
11:00				
4:00				
9:00				

M/S: Meal or Snack; H: Degree of Hunger (0 = None, 1 = Some, 2 = Normal, 3 = Good Healthy Hunger, 4 = Ravenous)

FOOD DIARY — Lesson Four

Day of Week ____________________ **Date** ____________________

Daily Activity Record Completed? yes___ no ___ Food Out of Sight? yes ___no ___

Time	M/S	H	Location of Eating	Comments
6:00				
11:00				
4:00				
9:00				

M/S: Meal or Snack; H: Degree of Hunger (0 = None, 1 = Some, 2 = Normal, 3 = Good Healthy Hunger, 4 = Ravenous)

FOOD DIARY — Lesson Four

Day of Week ______________________ Date ______________________

Daily Activity Record Completed? yes___ no___ Food Out of Sight? yes___no___

Time	M/S	H	Location of Eating	Comments
6:00				
11:00				
4:00				
9:00				

M/S: Meal or Snack; H: Degree of Hunger (0 = None, 1 = Some, 2 = Normal, 3 = Good Healthy Hunger, 4 = Ravenous)

FOOD DIARY — Lesson Four

Day of Week ____________________ Date ____________________

Daily Activity Record Completed? yes___ no___ Food Out of Sight? yes___ no___

Time	M/S	H	Location of Eating	Comments
6:00				
11:00				
4:00				
9:00				

M/S: Meal or Snack; H: Degree of Hunger (0 = None, 1 = Some, 2 = Normal, 3 = Good Healthy Hunger, 4 = Ravenous)

DAILY ACTIVITY RECORD

SAMPLE

(Fill in miles per day walked and minutes of exercise or extra activities)

	Monday		Tuesday		Wednesday		Thursday		Friday		Saturday		Sunday	
	Miles	Calories	Miles	Calories	Miles	Calories	Miles	Calories	Miles	Calories	Miles	Calories	Miles	Calories
Miles Walked	2½	350	3	420	2	280	3½	490	4	560	2	280	2½	315
Activity or Exercise	Mins.	Calories	Mins.	Calories	Mins.	Calories	Mins.	Calories	Mins.	Calories	Mins.	Calories	Mins.	Calories
BOWLING (ACTUAL ACTIVITY)			40	360										
GARDENING											30	141		
MOW LAWN (POWER)											40	212		
SWIMMING													20	126

Use the table on page 109 and 110 to calculate the caloric equivalent of each activity. If your activity is not included, chose one from the list that is similar.

DAILY ACTIVITY RECORD

(Fill in miles per day walked and minutes of exercise or extra activities)

	Monday		**Tuesday**		**Wednesday**		**Thursday**		**Friday**		**Saturday**		**Sunday**	
	Miles	**Calories**	**Miles**	**Calories**	**Miles**	**Calories**	**Miles**	**Calories**	**Miles**	**Calories**	**Miles**	**Calories**	**Miles**	**Calories**
Miles Walked														
Activity or Exercise	**Mins.**	**Calories**	**Mins.**	**Calories**	**Mins.**	**Calories**	**Mins.**	**Calories**	**Mins.**	**Calories**	**Mins.**	**Calories**	**Mins.**	**Calories**

Use the table on page 109 and 110 to calculate the caloric equivalent of each activity. If your activity is not included,

LESSON FIVE

BEING ACTIVE, CONTINUED— FITNESS VERSUS FATNESS

WEIGH-IN AND HOMEWORK

Weigh yourself, and record the weight on the Personal Weight Record.

You've covered a lot of ground in the past 4 weeks. You started with self-monitoring and have progressed to increasing activity. Presumably, you've had some weight loss, an increase in your overall level of activity, and some behavioral change.

REVIEW

Let's briefly review.

- Are you still self-monitoring? Yes ______ No ______
- Do your hunger ratings on your diaries reflect any change in your degree of hunger? Yes ______ No ______
- Has the number of places where you eat decreased, as reflected on your Eating Place Record? Yes ______ No ______
- Have you produced a snack-food-free environment? Yes ______ No ______

- Are you free of some of the "cues" that led you to extra eating in the past? Yes ______ No ______

- How have you dealt with those cues? ______________________

  ____

- Is the food in your home stored out of sight? Yes ______ No ______

- When eating do you only eat? Yes ______ No ______

- Have you changed your habitual eating place at the table? Yes ______ No ______ Once or twice? ______

- Have you taken the serving dishes from the table so you are less tempted to have seconds? Yes ______ No ______

Circle any areas that still need work. They will be part of this week's lesson.

Last week I talked about "tubbiness," and its relationship to exercise. What was true of Edward Bear is true for each of us. Inactivity often goes hand in hand with excess weight. More importantly, loss of weight must go hand in hand with an increase in activity.

In the near term you will accelerate your rate of weight loss and enhance your rate of metabolism. It is not only a tool to help you lose weight—good activity habits must be a permanent part of your daily lifestyle for "long-term weight control." Unfortunately, without a systematic activity program, almost 95% of people who lose weight regain it within six months.

- How many miles did you walk each day? Calculate it! I averaged ______ miles per day.

- How many minutes of non-routine activity or exercise did you do each day last week? ______

Last week I introduced the idea of an energy balance between calories consumed and calories burned up. We considered the equation:

ENERGY IN (food) = ENERGY USED (basal metabolism plus activity) + STORAGE (fat)

It can also be stated as follows:

STORAGE (fat) = ENERGY IN (food)
- ENERGY USED (basal metabolism plus activity)

This is a simplified form of one of the fundamental laws that governs the universe, the Second Law of Thermodynamics. There are no exceptions to this law, for man or beast.

During the first three lessons, this program concentrated on the "ENERGY IN" side of the equation. Much of your work to date has helped you reduce "ENERGY IN," by becoming more aware of your eating style through self monitoring, by slowing your eating to allow you to feel satiety or fullness, and by eliminating cues to inappropriate eating. By reducing the "ENERGY IN" side of the equation, you tipped the balanced towards the "ENERGY USED" side. You haven't taken in as much energy, and as a result some of your stored energy (fat) has been burned up.

Last week you learned that the "ENERGY USED" side of the equation is very important, and that it can work very effectively with reduced food intake to cause weight loss. Often an increase in exercise will reestablish the downward trend when you have reached a plateau where you feel stymied about continued weight loss. At other times a modest addition of exercise or activity to a weight control program can accelerate your rate of weight loss.

ENERGY: PART TWO

Most people are not aware of the amount of exercise or activity they engage in each day, or its effect on their weight. One study of obese housewives found that they spent more of their time in light activities such as sleeping, sitting, and watching television than a matched group of thin women. The thin subjects used one-sixth more energy during the day than the overweight women, despite the fact that overweight people use more calories per movement because of the extra work involved in moving their extra weight. (6)

Common sense tells us that if we exercise more we will become more hungry. This is true within a "natural" range of activities for most animals, including humans. But in a way we no longer live in a "natural" state. In the natural state, or even 50 years ago in our civilized society, people were more physically active than we are today. Now the average American spends much of his life sitting, or in other sedentary activities. We are the most efficient people in the history of the world—and we show it!

We are no longer operating in our "natural" activity range, and we are suffering from the same phenomenon that ranchers exploit when they put cattle in a feedlot. When penned up with excess food available, a steer eats more, becomes fat and less mobile, exercises less, gains weight and eats still more. It is a vicious cycle.

Several studies have shown that humans who adopt a sedentary lifestyle increase their food intake—just like cattle in a feedlot. (7) Conversely, when sedentary desk-bound people become more active—for example, when they change to a more active job—they eat less, and they lose weight.

Seven bonuses can be gained by working on the "ENERGY USED" (or increased activity) side of the energy equation:

1. If you incorporate exercise into your daily routine, a higher proportion of the weight you lose will come from fat deposits, the energy your body has stored as fat.
2. Some form of exertion or activity added to a dull routine can relieve some of the boredom (or blues) that frequently stimulates eating.
3. Strenuous exercise has a specific effect on appetite, particularly if you exercise hard before a meal. Frequently it will decrease your appetite.
4. As you lose weight, your body will regain a thin athletic shape.
5. Your body tone will improve, and your cardiovascular system will regain its ability to respond rapidly to stress and exercise.
6. You will enjoy life more.
7. Last, and perhaps most important, exercise may be one of the few ways of lowering your set point. This is important now, but it will be even more important once your weight is where you want it. Unless you can lower your set point, your body will always want to gain your weight back—and you will be hungry until it does! To escape this common fate, regular exercise and an increase in general activity must be part of your lifestyle from now on.

Before we go too far with a discussion of expending more energy by increasing activity, we need to look at some basic calculations and arrive at a feeling for what exercise calories mean—where all of that energy goes.

1. Energy is necessary to keep your body alive, to maintain vital functions: heart beat, breathing, body temperature, muscle tone, etc. The actual amount needed, the Basal Metabolic Rate (BMR), or resting energy expenditure, is affected by many factors: You burn more energy (have a higher metabolic rate) with increased surface area, fevers (14 percent elevation in BMR for each degree centigrade of fever), pregnancy, thyroid disease, and anxiety. Metabolic rates and food requirements are lower for old people, Chinese, Indians, individuals who are starved for a long time, and people who are depressed. The BMR is lower for women than for men.

   But regardless of an individual's metabolic rate, the laws of thermodynamics and the Energy Equation will hold true. A low BMR simply means you will have to lower your food intake below the point where people with a higher metabolic rate experience a weight loss; you need less energy (food) to stay at a constant weight, and you need still less to lose weight. It is not fair—your best friend, the same size and weight, may be able to eat more than you, yet still maintain her weight because her rate of metabolism is higher than yours. Every overweight person has had to live with this injustice of life.

2. Energy is used to digest food. Digesting proteins requires more calories than digesting fats, but the total amount of energy consumed in the digestion ("the specific dynamic action") is low, regardless of food type—less than seven percent of your total energy intake. (Claims that all protein calories are burned up in digestion are nonsense.)

3. All physical activity uses up energy. Sitting increases energy expenditure over lying down, and standing increases it even more—of course, exercise increases it further.

4. Energy is stored when you consume more than you burn. The storage is in that ugly stuff called fat.

How many calories do you need each day and how many calories should you eat if you want to lose weight? The simplest approximation is found in tables like Figure 3 . This data is for the "average-weight" American. Occupation, activity level, physical conditioning, body size, and other factors influencing Basal Metabolic Rate are *not* included in this table.

(Another very rough way to estimate your maintenance caloric requirement is to multiply your body weight by 10-13. For example, if you weigh 200 pounds, the approximate number of calories needed to

Figure 3 Mean Heights and Weights and Recommended Energy Intake. Food and Nutrition Board, National Academy of Sciences -- National Research Council, Ninth Edition.

	Age (years)	Weight (lbs)	Height (in.)	Calories
Infants	0.0-0.5	13	24	kg x 115
	0.5-1.0	20	28	kg x 105
Children	1-3	29	35	1300
	4-6	44	44	1700
	7-10	62	52	2400
Males	11-14	99	62	2700
	15-18	145	69	2800
	19-22	154	70	2900
	23-50	154	70	2700
	51-75	154	70	2400
	76+	154	70	2050
Females	11-14	101	62	2200
	15-18	120	64	2100
	19-22	120	64	2100
	23-50	120	64	2000
	51-75	120	64	1800
	76+	120	64	1600
Pregnant				+300
Lactation				+500

maintain your body weight is 2000-2600 calories per day. (200 x 10 = 2000 calories; 200 x 13 = 2600 calories.) Assuming you are only moderately active, to lose weight your caloric intake must be below this range. If you are relatively inactive, or are affected by any of a number of negative factors—like a recent starvation diet, or old age—that lower your resting energy needs, your caloric need for weight maintenance will probably be significantly below the range you get with this calculation.)

Remember, every table and calorie calculation is *approximate.* It doesn't matter what your exact caloric need is—for weight loss calculations what is important is consistency. The only way to determine *your* need is to progressively decrease your intake (and/or increase your activity level) until you are steadily losing weight. Remember too, as your weight drops, your daily caloric need also drops—there is less of you to feed.

Another general fact is that one pound of body fat is equal to a stored excess intake of 3500 calories. Thus a daily reduction of 500 calories below your daily caloric needs for maintenance of body weight will cause you to lose one pound a week. (500 calories x 7 days = 3500 calories.)

There are many refinements and correction factors that would have to be provided for if the calculation were to accurately predict exactly how much a pound of your weight is worth in calories. Even the best figures (calculated by measuring your carbon dioxide production at rest) are not entirely accurate. These rough guides have a potential error of up to 25 percent; nevertheless they are close enough to allow us to meaningfully discuss the energy values of different activities.

The absolute values for caloric expenditure you calculate today will be interesting. But they are only important if you are able to take advantage of what you learn, to change both your energy intake and you energy expenditure. More important than the absolute value of any of these calculations is the *relative* value in practice—that is, how much you can make them change.

Is This Clear So Far?

- Do you have any questions about the theory of energy balance or the Energy Equation? Yes ______ No ______ (pp. 74, 88)
- Do you understand where the energy goes that you consume in the form of food? Yes ______ No ______
- Did you get confused by the discussion of how to calculate the

number of calories you need each day to maintain your current weight? Yes ______ No ______ (page 91)

Keep in mind the fact that one pound of fat is the equivalent of 3500 calories:

–3500 taken in *beyond* the amount needed to maintain your body weight when you gain a pound;

–3500 calories burned off *beyond* what is taken in if you are to lose a pound.

Increasing Energy Expenditure

The lesson today deals with a sort of heresy—how to systematically *waste* energy and be inefficient. I want you to learn how to expend more effort and burn up more calories in the course of your routine daily activities.

The quickest way to burn up calories is to make large, fast movements, using as many large muscles as possible. This is why sports like swimming, tennis, cross country skiing, cycling, and jogging are good exercise. However, activities like these are not always possible, available, appropriate, or in your price range. And you may find them unpleasant. If you are like most people, you won't stick with anything for long if it is unpleasant. As least at the start, less strenuous increases will probably be more effective, because you will be more likely to stick with them.

There are two ways to increase your energy expenditure:

1. Increase your normal activities by becoming less efficient. Ask yourself the following question before you expend a single calorie: "Is this the most energetic or wasteful way I can do this?" When possible, sit instead of lie, stand instead of sit, take stairs instead of elevators, and walk instead of ride.
2. Introduce specific exercises, or increased activity, into your daily schedule.

During the next two or three weeks you should find that you can easily increase your evergy expenditure by 250 calories a day, by being both wasteful and energetic. In fact, some people can jump right in and add 250 extra calories of daily activity the first week. However, for most people, this, like all changes, will be difficult at first, and should probably be approached in steps of 50-100 calories per day each week. This will be easy if you are able to start a systematic daily exercise program.

Remember, when you are able to expend 250 calories worth of extra exercise every day, you will be rewarded with an extra half pound of weight loss each week (26 extra pounds in a year).

HOMEWORK

First, increase your daily activity by becoming less efficient. To give yourself information about your increase in activity continue to wear your pedometer and record the number of miles you walk each day. During the coming week try to walk 50 percent more miles each day than last week. For example, if you have been walking three miles a day, increase your daily mileage to four and a half miles next week. (3 miles + 1-1/2 miles = 4-1/2 miles.) The following are some ways to build an increase in walking into your everyday routine:

1. Answer the phone farthest away (but still close enough to get it before the ringing stops). If you have to get up to answer it, good; that is the best part. The phone company estimates that an extension phone saves you 70 miles a year of walking. (8) This is equivalent to 20 pounds in ten years. Avoid the 20 lbs.—and answer the extension that is farthest away.
2. Use the farthest bathroom at home and at work.
3. Park the car at the far end of the parking lot or an extra block from the store or your appointment. Choose the long way of walking places. (Leave a little early so you get there on time.) You will eventually enjoy these walks as a brief "time out."
4. Use stairs instead of elevators.
5. Stand as much as possible.
6. Walk rather than drive whenever possible.
7. Meet the bus at the next station down the line.

Be creative about ways to expend more energy. Extra activity becomes more enjoyable with time, practice, and mastery. Just as lethargy can become a habit, so can activity. When it becomes as automatic as brushing your teeth, you will have acquired a tremendously powerful weight loss maintenance tool.

Do These Ideas Get You Thinking About Extra Activity?

- Do you see how to use these hints to increase your walking next week?
  Yes ______ No ______

- Can you think of additional ways to walk farther during the day?
  1 ______________________________
  2 ______________________________
  3 ______________________________

Remember to record your additional mileage at the end of each day.

The second part of today's assignment is to increase the calories you expend in exercise. The easiest way to do this is to follow these guidelines:

1. Choose something you like to do, either a sport or more routine activity. Exercise does not have to be strenuous—some examples are gardening, easy jogging, and walking around the block.
2. Be sensible; start slowly and avoid strains that can catapult you back to a sitting (or lying) position.
3. Try to plan exercise ahead and to get a partner (for company and so that the temptation to avoid your exercise at the last moment is reduced). Most people find it easier and more enjoyable to exercise if they are with someone else, whether it is jogging or sex.
4. Choose active sports.

Record the number of minutes you spend exercising or in special activities on your Daily Activity Record. The materials for this lesson include a list of the approximate caloric values of various activities. Make a rough estimate of the number of calories you spend each day in physical activity other than walking, and try to increase it week by week. The more you burn up, the faster you will lose. Make exercise one of your new habits—it's worth it.

When you are doing the calculations today, remember, you are interested in the *amount of change* in your activity level between weeks, not in the absolute amount of exercises you are able to write down or the absolute number of calories calculated down to the last decimal point. This is not a race against anyone. If you try too hard and pull a muscle, it could backfire—take it easy at first, a small step at a time, and work into a good, regular program.

Do You Understand?

- If you do not understand the value of increased activity, the concept of increased energy expenditure with exercise, or your need for more activity, re-read pages 89–94.

A graph of calories expended in walking and other exercise will serve as feedback to let you know if you are burning up more calories this week than last week. Figure out your activity and energy expenditure for last week, fill in the "calories" on your Daily Activity Record, and plot the number of miles per day you walked last week on your Daily Energy Out (activity) Graph. This will be your baseline. Next week you will add to it to see how well you have been able to increase the energy-out (activity) side of the equation.

The homework assignment for this week is:

A. Lesson Five Food Diary

B. Daily Activity Record

C. Daily Energy-Out (activity) Graph

D. Complete the Eating Place Record (page 64, Lesson 3)

(Looking ahead to Lesson Nine, you will need a calorie counter or book that lists the caloric value of various foods. You may find a listing in one of your cookbooks. They can also be purchased at any bookstore and in many food markets and drug stores, or by sending one dollar to the Superintendent of Documents, U.S. Government Printing Office, Washington, D.C. 20402, and asking for Agriculture Information Bulletin No. 364, "Calories and Weight.")

FOOD DIARY — Lesson Five Sample

Day of Week Monday Date ________

Daily Activity Record Completed? yes ✓ no ___

Time	M/S	H	Location of Eating	Comments
6:00				
7:00	m	3	Kitchen	
10:00	S	0	Cafeteria	Skipped donuts at break
11:00				
12:30	M	S	Restaurant	
4:00				
4:45	S	0	Cafeteria	Needed energy— sweet roll and extra sugar in coffee
6:30	M	0	Dining Room	
9:00				
9:15	S	0	T.V. Room	Diet Soda

M/S: Meal or Snack; H: Degree of Hunger (0 = None, 1 = Some, 2 = Normal, 3 = Good Healthy Hunger, 4 = Ravenous)

FOOD DIARY — Lesson Five

Day of Week ____________________ Date ____________________

Daily Activity Record Completed? yes___ no ___

Time	M/S	H	Location of Eating	Comments
6:00				
11:00				
4:00				
9:00				

M/S: Meal or Snack; H: Degree of Hunger (0 = None, 1 = Some, 2 = Normal, 3 = Good Healthy Hunger, 4 = Ravenous)

FOOD DIARY — Lesson Five

Day of Week____________________ Date____________________

Daily Activity Record Completed? yes___ no ___

Time	M/S	H	Location of Eating	Comments
6:00				
11:00				
4:00				
9:00				

M/S: Meal or Snack; H: Degree of Hunger (0 = None, 1 = Some, 2 = Normal, 3 = Good Healthy Hunger, 4 = Ravenous)

FOOD DIARY — Lesson Five

Day of Week ______________________ Date ______________________

Daily Activity Record Completed? yes___ no ___

Time	M/S	H	Location of Eating	Comments
6:00				
11:00				
4:00				
9:00				

M/S: Meal or Snack; H: Degree of Hunger (0 = None, 1 = Some, 2 = Normal, 3 = Good Healthy Hunger, 4 = Ravenous)

FOOD DIARY — Lesson Five

Day of Week ____________________ Date ____________________

Daily Activity Record Completed? yes___ no ___

Time	M/S	H	Location of Eating	Comments
6:00				
11:00				
4:00				
9:00				

M/S: Meal or Snack; H: Degree of Hunger (0 = None, 1 = Some, 2 = Normal, 3 = Good Healthy Hunger, 4 = Ravenous)

FOOD DIARY — Lesson Five

Day of Week ________________ Date ________________

Daily Activity Record Completed? yes___ no ___

Time	M/S	H	Location of Eating	Comments
6:00				
11:00				
4:00				
9:00				

M/S: Meal or Snack; H: Degree of Hunger (0 = None, 1 = Some, 2 = Normal, 3 = Good Healthy Hunger, 4 = Ravenous)

FOOD DIARY — Lesson Five

Day of Week____________________ Date____________________

Daily Activity Record Completed? yes___ no ___

Time	M/S	H	Location of Eating	Comments
6:00				
11:00				
4:00				
9:00				

M/S: Meal or Snack; H: Degree of Hunger (0 = None, 1 = Some, 2 = Normal, 3 = Good Healthy Hunger, 4 = Ravenous)

FOOD DIARY — Lesson Five

Day of Week ____________________ Date ____________________

Daily Activity Record Completed? yes___ no ___

Time	M/S	H	Location of Eating	Comments
6:00				
11:00				
4:00				
9:00				

M/S: Meal or Snack; H: Degree of Hunger (0 = None, 1 = Some, 2 = Normal, 3 = Good Healthy Hunger, 4 = Ravenous)

DAILY ACTIVITY RECORD

(Fill in miles per day walked and minutes of exercise or extra activities)

	Monday		Tuesday		Wednesday		Thursday		Friday		Saturday		Sunday	
	Miles	Calories	Miles	Calories	Miles	Calories	Miles	Calories	Miles	Calories	Miles	Calories	Miles	Calories
Miles Walked														
Activity or Exercise	Mins.	Calories	Mins.	Calories	Mins.	Calories	Mins.	Calories	Mins.	Calories	Mins.	Calories	Mins.	Calories

Use the table on page 109 and 110 to calculate the caloric equivalent of each activity. If your activity is not included, chose one from the list that is similar.

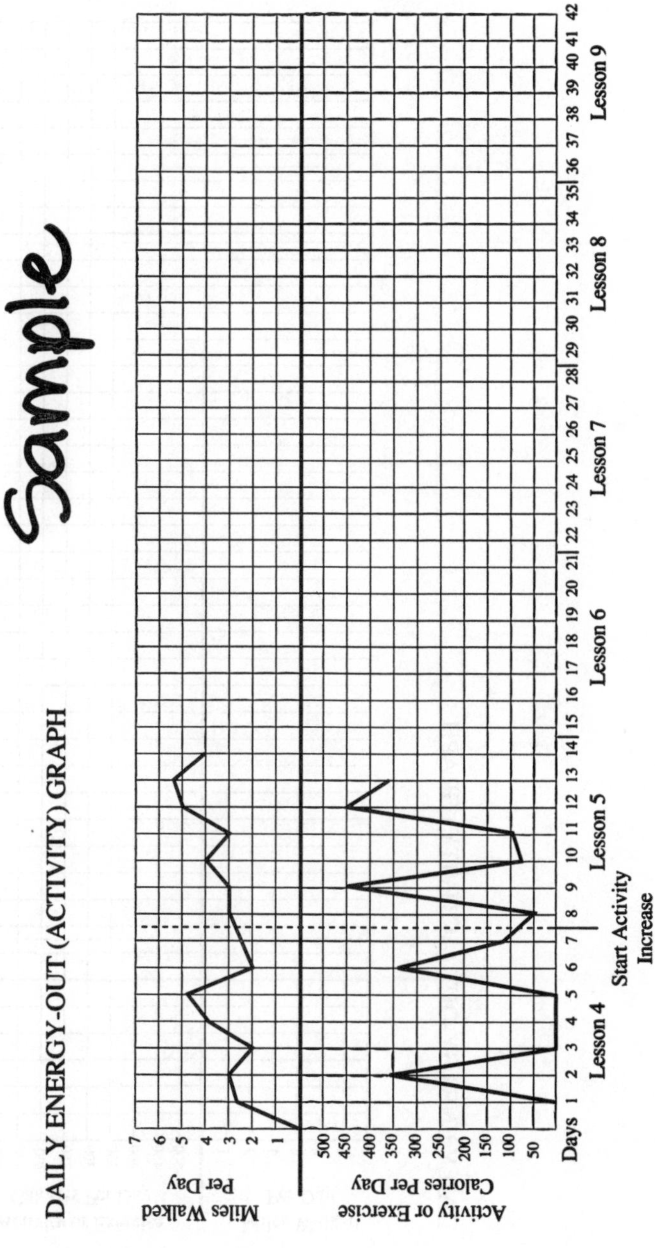
Sample
DAILY ENERGY-OUT (ACTIVITY) GRAPH
Miles Walked Per Day
7
6
5
4
3
2
1
Activity or Exercise Calories Per Day
500
450
400
350
300
250
200
150
100
50
Days 1 2 3 4 5 6 7 8 9 10 11 12 13 14 15 16 17 18 19 20 21 22 23 24 25 26 27 28 29 30 31 32 33 34 35 36 37 38 39 40 41 42
Lesson 4
Start Activity Increase
Lesson 5
Lesson 6
Lesson 7
Lesson 8
Lesson 9

DAILY ENERGY-OUT (ACTIVITY) GRAPH

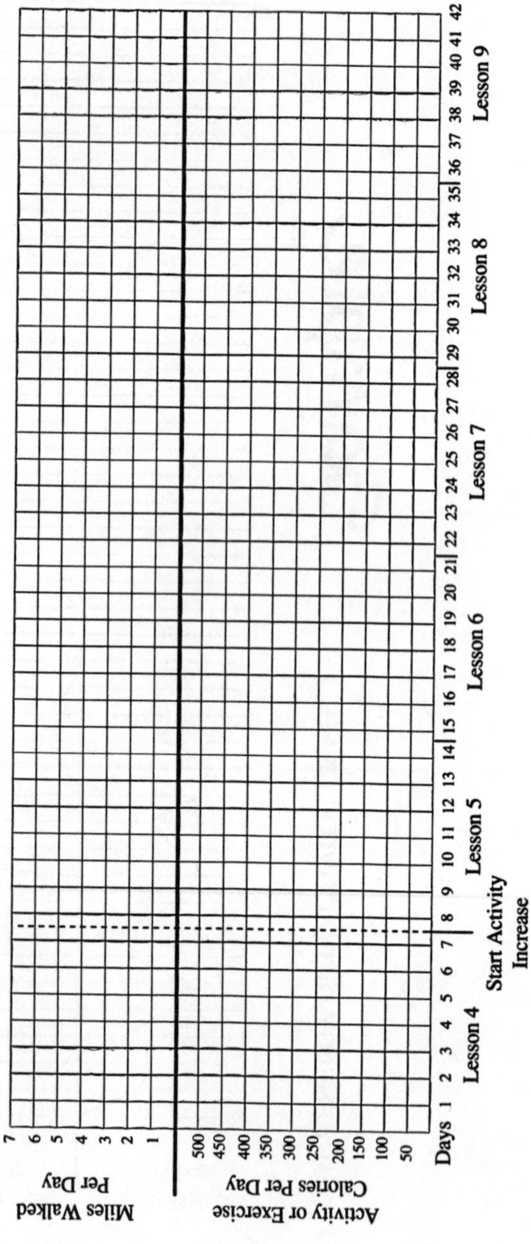

CALORIES BURNED UP DURING TEN MINUTES OF CONTINUOUS ACTIVITY

	Body Wt.#	150#	175#	200#	225#	250#	275#	300#
LOCOMOTION								
Walking - 2 mph		35	40	46	53	58	64	69
One mile - @ 2 mph		105	120	140	157	175	193	210
Walking - 4-1/2 mph		67	78	87	98	110	120	131
One mile - @ 4-1/2 mph		89	103	115	130	147	160	173
Walking Upstairs		175	201	229	259	288	318	350
Walking Downstairs		67	78	88	100	111	122	134
Jogging - 5-1/2 mph		108	127	142	160	178	197	215
Running - 7 mph		141	164	187	208	232	256	280
Running - 12 mph (sprint)		197	230	258	295	326	360	395
Running in place (140 count)		242	284	325	363	405	447	490
Bicycle - 5-1/2 mph		50	58	67	75	83	92	101
Bicycle - 13 mph		107	125	142	160	178	197	216
RECREATION								
Badminton or Vollyball		52	67	75	85	94	104	115
Baseball (except pitcher)		47	54	62	70	78	86	94
Basketball		70	82	93	105	117	128	140
Bowling (nonstop)		67	82	90	100	111	122	133
Canadian Airforce								
Exercise -0.5 Bx 1A		83	97	108	123	137	152	168
2A		104	122	137	155	173	190	207
3A,4A		147	170	192	217	244	267	290
5A,6A		167	192	217	240	270	300	330
Dancing - moderate		42	49	55	62	69	77	86
Dancing - vigorous		57	67	75	86	94	104	115
Square Dancing		68	80	90	103	113	124	135
Football		83	97	110	123	137	152	167
Golf - foursome		40	47	55	62	68	75	83
Horseback Riding (trot)		67	78	90	102	112	123	134
Ping Pong		38	43	52	58	64	71	78
Skiing - (alpine)		96	113	128	145	160	177	195
Skiing - (cross country)		117	137	158	174	194	214	235
Skiing - (water)		73	92	104	117	130	142	165
Swimming - (backstroke) 20 yd/min		38	43	52	58	64	71	79
Swimming - (breaststroke) 20 yd/min		48	55	63	72	80	88	96
Swimming - crawl 20 yd/min		48	55	63	72	80	88	96
Tennis		67	80	92	103	115	125	135
Wrestling, Judo or Karate		129	150	175	192	213	235	257

CALORIES BURNED UP DURING TEN MINUTES OF CONTINUOUS ACTIVITY (Continued)

	Body Wt.#	150#	175#	200#	225#	250#	275#	300#
PERSONAL ACTIVITIES								
Sleeping		12	14	16	18	20	22	24
Sitting (TV or reading)		12	14	16	18	20	22	24
Sitting (Conversing)		18	21	24	28	30	34	37
Washing/Dressing		32	38	42	47	53	58	63
Standing quietly		14	17	19	21	24	26	28
SEDENTARY OCCUPATION								
Sitting/Writing		18	21	24	28	30	34	37
Light Office Work		30	35	39	45	50	55	60
Standing (Light activity)		24	28	32	37	40	45	50
HOUSEWORK								
General Housework		41	48	53	60	68	74	81
Washing Windows		42	49	54	61	69	76	83
Making Beds		39	46	52	58	65	75	85
Mopping Floors		46	54	60	68	75	83	91
Light Gardening		36	42	47	53	59	66	73
Weeding Garden		59	69	78	88	98	109	120
Mowing Grass (power)		41	48	53	60	67	74	81
Mowing Grass (manual)		45	53	58	66	74	81	88
Shoveling Snow		78	92	100	117	130	144	160
LIGHT WORK								
Factory Assembly		24	28	32	37	40	45	50
Truck-Auto Repair		42	49	54	61	69	76	83
Carpentry/Farm Work		38	45	51	58	64	71	78
Brick Laying		34	40	45	51	57	62	67
HEAVY WORK								
Chopping Wood		73	86	96	109	121	134	156
Pick & Shovel Work		67	79	88	100	110	120	130

LESSON SIX

MAINTENANCE— KEYS FOR SURVIVAL

WEIGH-IN

Weigh yourself and record the weight on the Personal Weight Record as you have done each week. Graph your weight, and see how close you are to the average weight loss printed on the form. How are you doing? What is your total weight loss?______

Check your homework from Lesson Five.

- Is your food diary complete? Yes______ No______
- Have you noticed any trends? Yes______ No______
- Are you eating fewer snacks? Yes______ No______
- When you do snack, are you a little hungry or not hungry at all? Yes______ No______
- Is there any trend in the location of your eating? Yes______ No______
- Did you keep track of your daily activities and exercise this week? Yes______ No______
- Did you complete the Eating Place Record (Lesson Three, page 64)? Yes______ No______
- Did your Appropriately Designated Eating Place become your usual eating location? Yes______ No______

REVIEW

We have emphasized energy use for the last 2 weeks. You were asked to chart the miles per day that you walked this last week, and the amount of activity or exercise in addition to your usual daily activity. Then you graphed this on your Daily Activity Chart.

- Have you seen any trends in this? Yes______ No______
- How does it compare with the baseline that you graphed last week? greater______ less______ the same______

You can calculate the calories you've burned up by using the table on pages 109–110. It's amazing how much energy can be expended in simple everyday activities. Modest activities like making beds, weeding the garden, and washing windows add up in the same way as heavy work like chopping wood, and digging trenches in the back yard. Remember, if you're overweight and out of shape, take it easy. Work up to that wood pile by engaging in some lighter activities first.

It will be a while before the extra benefits of increased activity begin to show up. With time your cardiovascular system will be stronger, your muscles will be more firm, and you will begin to feel good—and more in control of your body.

NEW TECHNIQUE: MAINTENANCE

You've been at it for five continuous weeks. You've been losing weight, increasing your activity, limiting the places at which you eat, and becoming much more aware of the many little habits that contribute to excessive weight. You've changed the place where you eat, the places you store food, and the activities that accompany your eating.

It's time to take a break!

This next week is for practice, or maintenance. Of all the principles in the behavioral treatment of weight control, the most important is maintenance.

You can lose weight by locking yourself in the closet for a month with no food. This is a guaranteed, sure-fire way to lose pounds and inches. The problem with it is that it teaches you nothing. You would endure all of the gloom and darkness of a closet, only to emerge ravenously hungry, and go back to your old habits (after an extensive eating binge). Maintenance, and the practice of maintenance are the keys to long-term weight control.

For the next week I have provided a Daily Behavior Checklist. On it I want you to check each of the listed behavioral tasks when you do them. In the evening after dinner, rate yourself on a scale from 1 to 3 to judge how well you've been able to practice the behaviors you've learned during the first 5 weeks.

During this week it's particularly important to keep active. Continue to fill out your Daily Activity Record. When you have recorded your miles walked and calories of extra activity expended for the day, turn back to Lesson Five, p. 108, and plot the numbers on the Energy-Out (activity) Graph, for Lesson Six.

Do not jump ahead to the next lesson. Although maintenance may seem like vacation, it is not only spelled differently, but has a radically different meaning. There is no point in losing weight unless you are resolved to maintain that weight loss *forever*.

DAILY BEHAVIOR CHECKLIST — Lesson Six

Sample

Points: Most of the time, or yes =3
Sometimes =2
Not at all, no =1

	Days of the Week						
	1	2	3	4	5	6	7
1. *Daily Checklist* a. Morning review of anticipated eating	3	3	3	3	3	3	3
b. Evening recording of what was eaten	3	3	3	3	3	3	3
2. *Food Diary* - make one only with items that you feel will help (like recording just degree of hunger or times you snacked).	2	3	3	3	3	3	2
3. *Cue Elimination* a. Designated eating place	2	3	2	3	3	3	1
b. Food stored in opaque containers	2	2	2	3	3	3	3
4. *Energy Use* a. Record miles walked per day	2	2	2	3	2	2	2
b. Increase in miles walked per day	2	2	2	3	2	3	1
c. Increase minutes of other activities	2	1	2	2	1	2	2
DAILY TOTALS	18	19	19	23	20	22	17

Total Points for the Week 138   Weight ________

DAILY BEHAVIOR CHECKLIST — Lesson Six

Points: Most of the time, or yes =3
Sometimes =2
Not at all, no =1

	Days of the Week						
	1	2	3	4	5	6	7
1. *Daily Checklist* a. Morning review of anticipated eating							
b. Evening recording of what was eaten							
2. *Food Diary* - make one only with items that you feel will help (like recording just degree of hunger or times you snacked).							
3. *Cue Elimination* a. Designated eating place							
b. Food stored in opaque containers							
4. *Energy Use* a. Record miles walked per day							
b. Increase in miles walked per day							
c. Increase minutes of other activities							
DAILY TOTALS							

Total Points for the Week ___________ Weight _________

DAILY ACTIVITY RECORD

(Fill in miles per day walked and minutes of exercise or extra activities)

	Monday		**Tuesday**		**Wednesday**		**Thursday**		**Friday**		**Saturday**		**Sunday**	
	Miles	**Calories**	**Miles**	**Calories**	**Miles**	**Calories**	**Miles**	**Calories**	**Miles**	**Calories**	**Miles**	**Calories**	**Miles**	**Calories**
Miles Walked														
Activity or Exercise	**Mins.**	**Calories**	**Mins.**	**Calories**	**Mins.**	**Calories**	**Mins.**	**Calories**	**Mins.**	**Calories**	**Mins.**	**Calories**	**Mins.**	**Calories**

Use the table on page 109 and 110 to calculate the caloric equivalent of each activity. If your activity is not included, chose one from the list that is similar

LESSON SEVEN

BEHAVIOR CHAINS AND ALTERNATE ACTIVITIES— ONE THING LEADS TO ANOTHER

WEIGH-IN AND HOMEWORK

Weigh yourself and record the change for the week on your Personal Weight Record.

My total weight loss for the past 6 weeks is______.

Using the calories of extra activity and miles walked recorded on your Lesson Six Daily Activity Record, graph the calories burned and miles walked on your Energy-Out (activity) Graph (p. 108) for Lesson Six.

REVIEW

Last week was your first maintenance week. In a program like this, practice makes the difference between success and failure. Maintenance, or practice weeks, will be included periodically to give you time to practice, and to avoid the feeling of being overwhelmed. One member of a weight loss program compared this course to juggling. The first ball, and the next few additional balls are easy to control, provided you don't take them on too quickly. At some point, however, if you add just one more too soon, they all fall to the ground.

Prior to this week we covered a wide number of behavioral techniques. These included awareness exercises, using food diaries to help you become aware of the multitude of tiny habits that accompa ny your excess eating. Some of the lessons included not eating when you are not really hungry, not eating when standing or doing other activities that might distract you from your food, not eating in inappropriate places, and identifying the way you eat in response to a variety of food cues.

You looked at your home eating, snacking, and food storage, and went through a "home decalorization" process. All the extra food around the house was gathered up, taken to the kitchen, and either thrown away or stored out of sight. Snacks were moved to more appropriate places—or eliminated altogether.

- Are you still keeping all food in the kitchen? Or has it crept back to it's hiding places around the house?
  Yes______ No______

I talked about the small cues or stimuli in the environment that turn on our desire to eat even when our bodies aren't hungry. You learned that you could actually affect the amount you eat, by learning how to get rid of these cues with specific techniques. These techniques, collectively referred to as stimulus control or cue elimination, took a variety of forms, concluding with six "commandments":

I. Choose a specific place to eat.

II. Change your habitual eating place at the table.

III. When eating, only eat.

IV. Remove food from all non-food places in the house.

V. Replace junk or convenience food with foods of low-caloric density.

VI. Do not keep serving containers on the table.

These sound simple, but in practice most people find them difficult. They increase your awareness of your eating patterns and habits, and they decrease the probability of excess nibbling.

- Are you still continuing with these exercises?
  Yes______ No______
- Circle the three that have helped you the most.

Activity is vital to weight loss. Lessons 4 and 5 dealt with this in detail. Initially you made a baseline measurement of your miles walked per day, and minutes per day of extra activity. Then you increased your miles per day, and tried to increase your energy expenditure by being more active. Techniques for this included parking farther away from your destinations, standing when you could be sitting, using stairs instead of elevators, and using the phone at the other end of the house.

- Are you still making a conscious effort to waste energy?
  Yes______ No______
- Have you parked further away from a store this past week?
  Yes______ No______
- How many miles per day did you average walking during the maintenance period?______
- How many minutes of extra activity did you average during the past week?______
- How many calories did you burn up in exercise (walking + activity)?______
- During the maintenance week, you kept a Daily Behavior Checklist. Did you fill it out every day? Yes______ No______

If you think this checklist would be helpful as a reminder, make additional copies and fill them in over the next few weeks.

Turn back to Lesson Five (page 108) to the Daily Energy-Out (activity) Graph. Extend the graph to include the miles per day and calories per day of activities you recorded on the maintenance week Daily Behavior Checklist.

- Is there a trend upwards for miles per day walked?
  Yes______ No______
- Is there a trend upwards for calories per day expended in activities?
  Yes______ No______

NEW TECHNIQUE: BEHAVIOR CHAINS AND ALTERNATE ACTIVITIES

We are all creatures of habit. We repeat the same patterns of behavior over and over and over. Nowhere is this more true than with eating habits.

A typical behavior pattern for an over-eater businessman is to come home from work, put down his briefcase, pick up the paper, sit down and turn on the television, get up and look in the refrigerator, pick out a snack, sit back in front of the television, pick up the paper, eat, watch television, and when dinner is ready, have a meal. He might also finish his meal, sit down to watch TV, get bored, walk into the kitchen, browse through the refrigerator, eat a piece of cheescake, and wander back to the TV.

Although the specifics of the behavior may be different, the patterns are usually similar day after day after day. Similarly, we often find ourselves eating in situations where food might not be appropriate. In both types of cases, the chain of behaviors which leads to excess eating (or excess eating in response to something that's going on right now—for example, tension, stress or boredom) could be prevented if you are: (1) Aware of it; (2) If you have something else to do.

Look at this typical behavior chain. How many eating situations in your life can you describe with a similar diagram?

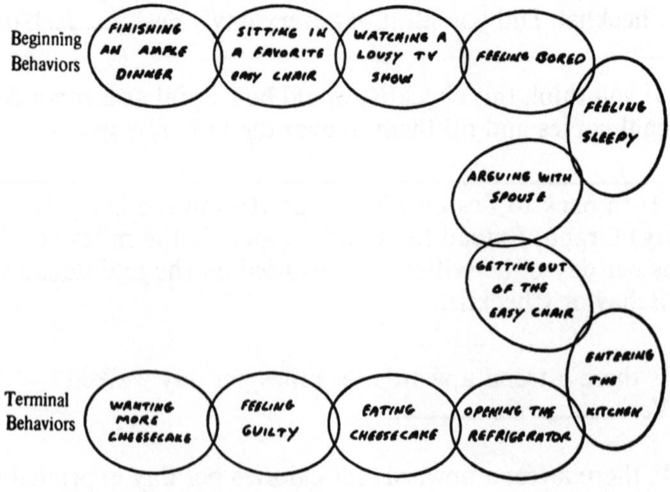

Looking at this series of linked events suggests a strategy for eliminating a great deal of extra, habitual eating or snacking. Break

the chain! The earlier in the chain, the better and the easier. Once that snack touches your taste buds, it's too late.

The principle behind activity substitution is quite simple. Behaviors occur in chains. Eating (or more precisely, feeling bad about eating) is at one end of a chain of responses. As you work backwards from the final behaviors, you can recognize events (or cues) in your environment that started the chain of events that led to eating.

Using activities to break up patterns of behaviors that lead to inappropriate eating can be a very powerful means of changing eating habits. This activity substitution technique is useful when you are eating in response to environmental as well as internal cues—for instance the hunger pangs you feel at odd times, like after meals, before bed, or when you are out shopping, or during periods of stress, boredom, or frustration.

The trick to substituting alternate activities for eating is to think in advance about what would be available, and/or appropriate. There are four types of behaviors that can be substituted for behavioral chains that lead to eating for inappropriate reasons:

First consider *fun* activities. For example, instead of watching the same boring TV show, take a walk and talk to the neighbors, or just look at the scenery.

Second, you can agree with yourself that when the occasion arises and you're headed toward the refrigerator, you'll have to do a *necessary* activity before eating. For example, clean up a room in the house, balance the checkbook, or take the car and get some gas.

Third, you can always combat the urge with an *incompatible* activity—for example, taking a shower. It's very hard to snack in the shower. By the time you're drying yourself off after your shower, the urge to eat has disappeared.

Fourth, if nothing else, *time consuming activities* will help you stave off extra eating. 90% of the time, if an urge is not responded to within 20 minutes it will go away. Most urges to eat are transient, partly because they are related to a stimulus in the environment that triggers the urge, which on closer examination, has no relationship to food.

Once the urge comes, set the kitchen timer for twenty minutes, and go on with your daily activities. When the timer rings, if you still feel like eating, go ahead and have a low-calorie snack. On the other hand, if you're not still hungry, you've conquered the urge.

If the chain is broken at any point, it probably will not continue, and the final behaviors in the chain, eating and feeling guilty, will not occur. The earlier in the chain you identify the trend towards eating, the easier it is to intervene. If you don't identify the chain until you have opened the refrigerator door, it may be too late.

The interventions can be very simple. Once the behavior chain has been identified, it is a matter of selecting an alternative activity that will either not progress toward eating, or will delay eating until your hunger has diminished.

In the above example, you may recognize that your favorite chair always leads to this chain of behaviors after dinner. Watching TV somewhere else may break the chain. A more stimulating TV show, or a copy of a sexy book, may help hold your attention and break the chain. If you feel bored and sleepy, a ten-minute nap may unlink the chain. A prior agreement with yourself to wash the dishes before having a snack might either save you from the dishwashing chore, or delay your eating until you are no longer hungry. If you got as far as the refrigerator, you could have a pre-prepared alternate snack of carrots or fruit to deter you from the left-over cheescake.

Finally, if you do eat the cheesecake, try not to feel guilty; you simply were not prepared to break the chain at this time.

Let's Consider This New Concept a Bit

- Do you understand the concept of behavior chains? Yes______ No______ (It is important that you do understand it. Re-read the last section if it is not absolutely clear.)

- Can you think of an example of a behavior chain that occurs in your life? Yes______ No______ (You will have a chance to fill one in when you do today's homework.)

- Do you see how breaking a chain like the sample one in this lesson can help you avoid inappropriate eating? Yes______ No______

- What would be the easiest link for you to break in this type of chain? Circle it and draw in a new link with an alternate activity that would steer you away from the eating you want to avoid.

If your hunger occurs at a fixed time each day, the links in the chain that lead to eating may not be obvious. The most direct strategy to overcome this hunger with its habitual snack is to substitute a non-food related activity for eating. For example, if you know you have a craving for food at 3:15 every afternoon, you can rearrange your schedule so you are engaged in an activity that is incompatible with eating between 2:45 and 3:45. You will be changing the terminal end of the behavior chain by substituting some other activity for your usual 3:15 snack.

Alternate activities could include walking the dog, playing tennis, taking a bath, washing your hair, or sleeping. *Hunger pangs are short-lived*, and if you delay eating for 10 or 15 minutes, the urge to eat will usually diminish.

The hunger you feel at odd times is probably a conditioned response to a cue in your environment, even though you are not able to identify it while you are responding to it. If feeling hungry is not rewarded with food, the hunger response will diminish with time. The unknown environmental cue will lose its ability to arouse your hunger.

All substitute activities must possess two important qualities: They must be readily available, and they must be able to compete with the urge to eat. Two types of activities can compete with hunger: (a) pleasant activities, and (b) necessary activities—things you have to do each day, hungry or not.

Some examples of pleasant substitutions are: a hobby, a walk around the block, working in the garden, reading a good book, listening to music, taking a leisurely bath, and sleeping. Some examples of the necessary type of activities are: errands, cleaning the house, doing homework, working on household projects, making phone calls, paying bills, washing the floor, and shopping. If possible the activity you choose should be incompatible with eating.

Re-Consider All of This for a Moment

- Do you understand what an alternate activity is?
  Yes______ No______

- Write down a pleasant activity that might be substituted for eating.

  ____

- Write down an activity that is incompatible with eating. (It may be one of the activities you thought of when we were considering "pleasant" and "necessary" activities.)

  ____

Remember, you are often trying to outwit a hunger pang that has a life expectancy of only 10 to 15 minutes.

A more neutral way to break a behavior chain, especially if you are aware of only the terminal behaviors (eating once in a while for no reason) is to add time between the links. This is easily accomplished by setting a cooking timer, parking meter, or alarm clock for a pre-set number of minutes, and delaying the snack.

At first, interpose five to ten minutes. Then gradually increase the time between the urge to snack and your actually eating to 15 to 20 minutes. While you are waiting to eat, do something else. You will be amazed at how few snacks you will want if you wait a few minutes between the time you first recognize an urge to eat and the point when you actually open the refrigerator door.

HOMEWORK

Identify at least one of your eating behavior chains. The homework forms include an Alternate Activity Sheet, which contains a blank chain. Start analyzing your behavior by selecting an eating situation that occurs fairly often during the week. This could be an afternoon snack, an urge for food in the morning, or a bite to eat while watching TV or studying in the evening. Write down when and where you find yourself eating, and try to fill in each step that precedes it. When you are done, it will look like our earlier example.

After you have defined a behavior chain, plan several alternate activities to break the chain at its weakest link. During the week record whether or not your chain-breaking strategies were successful.

If you can identify only the final link in a behavior chain, plan an alternate activity that will take the place of the eating response, or at least introduce a delay before you eat. The easiest way to make this technique work is to have a list of alternate activities prepared in advance, and introduce them between the urge to snack and the actual eating.

On the Alternate Activity Sheet you will find a place to record six alternate responses: three should be activities that are pleasant, that can compete with hunger just by being enjoyable, and three should be necessary activities that can compete because you are obligated to do them during the day.

Try to make a substitution every day. Write down each time you are successful in substituting an alternate response for eating.

One strategy that may be useful is to give yourself permission to snack at first, by saying to yourself something like, "I am hungry and I want a snack, but before I eat it, I will____________________."

A great deal of extra eating takes place when people are bored or fatigued. If you can prevent boredom, you may be able to prevent over-eating. Your Alternate Activity Sheet may be able to help you do this, by providing an easily accessible list of things to do when you are bored and can't think of anything to do.

If you find you are eating because of fatigue, then the appropriate response is a ten-minute nap rather than food. Sometimes it is hard to distinguish between boredom and fatigue—but a nap is not only non-caloric and incompatible with eating, it is also refreshing.

The homework assignment for this week is:

A. A simplified Food/Activity Diary.

B. A Daily Activity Record

C. An Alternate Activity Sheet. Write down one of your behavior chains on the Alternate Activity Sheet. Take a few minutes and think it over. Perhaps you will want to discuss it with your family. Regular chains of behaviors occur in all lives—we simply don't pay attention to them.

D. Plan an "unlinking strategy." Find the weak link in your eating behavior chain and plan an alternate activity to hook onto that weak link.

E. Keep track of the situations where you were able to break an eating chain.

FOOD ACTIVITY DIARY — Lesson Seven

Day of Week ____________________ Date ____________________

Time	M/S	H	Activity Increased yes/no	Miles Per Day Increased yes/no	Comments
6:00					
11:00					
4:00					
9:00					

M/S: Meal or Snack; H: Degree of Hunger (0 = None, 1 = Some, 2 = Normal, 3 = Good Healthy Hunger, 4 = Ravenous)

FOOD ACTIVITY DIARY — Lesson Seven

Day of Week ____________ Date ____________

Time	M/S	H	Activity Increased yes/no	Miles Per Day Increased yes/no	Comments
6:00					
11:00					
4:00					
9:00					

M/S: Meal or Snack; H: Degree of Hunger (0 = None, 1 = Some, 2 = Normal, 3 = Good Healthy Hunger, 4 = Ravenous)

FOOD ACTIVITY DIARY — Lesson Seven

Day of Week ____________________ Date ____________________

Time	M/S	H	Activity Increased yes/no	Miles Per Day Increased yes/no	Comments
6:00					
11:00					
4:00					
9:00					

M/S: Meal or Snack; H: Degree of Hunger (0 = None, 1 = Some, 2 = Normal, 3 = Good Healthy Hunger, 4 = Ravenous)

FOOD ACTIVITY DIARY — Lesson Seven

Day of Week ____________________ Date ____________________

Time	M/S	H	Activity Increased yes/no	Miles Per Day Increased yes/no	Comments
6:00					
11:00					
4:00					
9:00					

M/S: Meal or Snack; H: Degree of Hunger (0 = None, 1 = Some, 2 = Normal, 3 = Good Healthy Hunger, 4 = Ravenous)

FOOD ACTIVITY DIARY — Lesson Seven

Day of Week ______________ Date ______________

Time	M/S	H	Activity Increased yes/no	Miles Per Day Increased yes/no	Comments
6:00					
11:00					
4:00					
9:00					

M/S: Meal or Snack; H: Degree of Hunger (0 = None, 1 = Some, 2 = Normal, 3 = Good Healthy Hunger, 4 = Ravenous)

FOOD ACTIVITY DIARY — Lesson Seven

Day of Week ______________ Date ______________

Time	M/S	H	Activity Increased yes/no	Miles Per Day Increased yes/no	Comments
6:00					
11:00					
4:00					
9:00					

M/S: Meal or Snack; H: Degree of Hunger (0 = None, 1 = Some, 2 = Normal, 3 = Good Healthy Hunger, 4 = Ravenous)

FOOD ACTIVITY DIARY — Lesson Seven

Day of Week ______________________ Date ______________________

Time	M/S	H	Activity Increased yes/no	Miles Per Day Increased yes/no	Comments
6:00					
11:00					
4:00					
9:00					

M/S: Meal or Snack; H: Degree of Hunger (0 = None, 1 = Some, 2 = Normal, 3 = Good Healthy Hunger, 4 = Ravenous)

DAILY ACTIVITY RECORD

(Fill in miles per day walked and minutes of exercise or extra activities)

	Monday		Tuesday		Wednesday		Thursday		Friday		Saturday		Sunday	
	Miles	Calories	Miles	Calories	Miles	Calories	Miles	Calories	Miles	Calories	Miles	Calories	Miles	Calories
Miles Walked														
Activity or Exercise	Mins.	Calories	Mins.	Calories	Mins.	Calories	Mins.	Calories	Mins.	Calories	Mins.	Calories	Mins.	Calories

Use the table on page 109 and 110 to calculate the caloric equivalent of each activity. If your activity is not included, chose one from the list that is similar.

ALTERNATE ACTIVITY SHEET

SAMPLE

SUBSTITUTE ACTIVITIES

Pleasant Activities
1. SINGING - WASHING HAIR
2. PLAYING PIANO - BIKING
3. SEWING - CALLING "SHUT-INS"

Necessary Activities
1. DUSTING
2. VACUMMING
3. STRAIGHTEN HOUSE

Situations when used
1. WANTED ICE CREAM - DELAYED WITH BATH
2. WANTED WHEAT THINS - CLEANED UP YARD
3. WANTED SNACK - WENT FOR WALK
4. WANTED COOKIES - DID DISHES FIRST
5. SAW LEFT OVERS - THREW THEM OUT; WENT FOR BIKE RIDE
6. TEMPTED BY COOKIES - SET TIMER
7. WANTED SNACK - PLAYED PIANO

BEHAVIOR CHAIN

Identify the links in your eating response chain on the following diagram. Draw a line through the chain where it was interrupted. Add the link you substituted and the new chain of behaviors this substitution started.

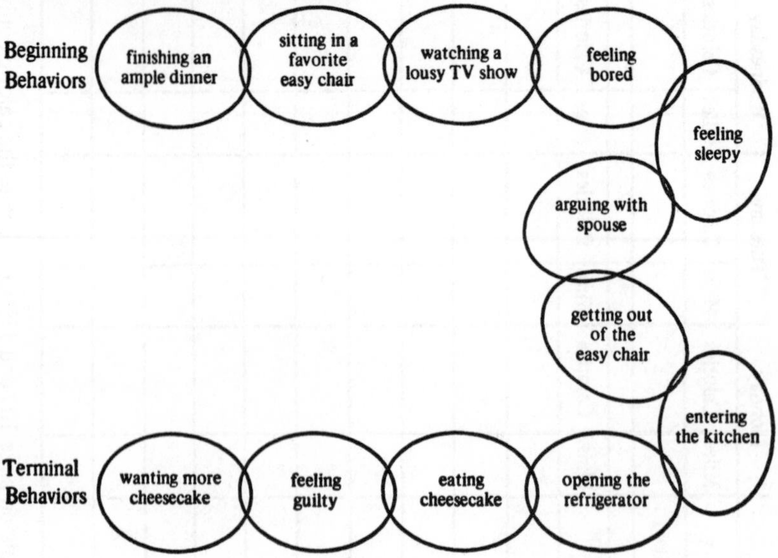

ALTERNATE ACTIVITY SHEET

SUBSTITUTE ACTIVITIES

Pleasant Activities
1. ______
2. ______
3. ______

Necessary Activities
1. ______
2. ______
3. ______

Situations when used
1. ______
2. ______
3. ______
4. ______
5. ______
6. ______
7. ______

BEHAVIOR CHAIN

Identify the links in your eating response chain on the following diagram. Draw a line through the chain where it was interrupted. Add the link you substituted and the new chain of behaviors this substitution started.

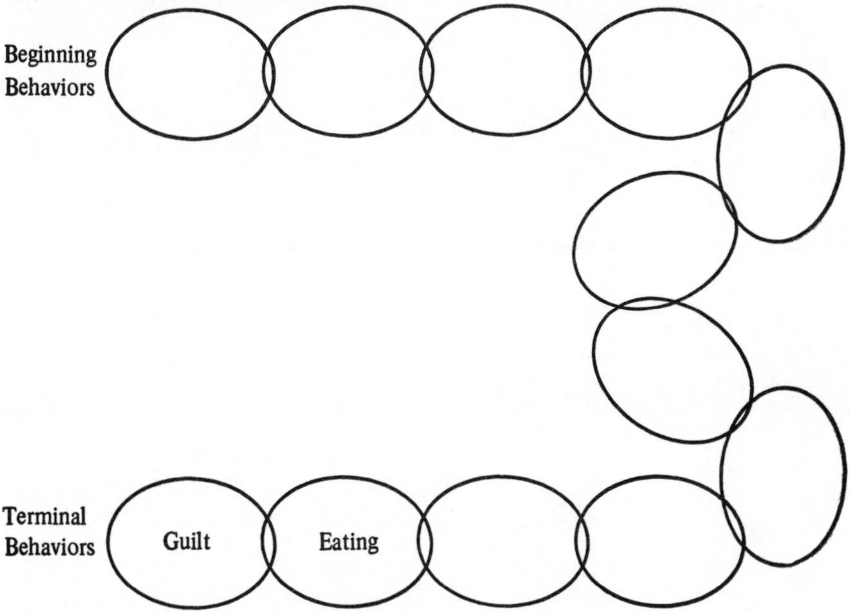

LESSON EIGHT

THE ACT: EATING— CHANGING YOUR STYLE

WEIGH-IN AND HOMEWORK

Weigh yourself and record your weight on your Personal Weight Record. Graph your weight change for the past week.

Compare your weight loss with the average weight loss line of one pound per week.

Check your homework.

- Is your Lesson Seven Food Diary and Daily Activity Record complete? Yes______ No______

- Add this week's miles and calories of activity to your Daily Energy-Out (activity) graph (p.108). Is the trend still upward? Yes______ No______

- Did you define a behavior chain and fill out your Alternate Activity Sheet? Yes______ No______

- Did you keep a record of situations where you were able to break a behavior chain? Yes______ No______

Give yourself credit towards your refund on your Homework Credit Sheet. If your activity level is still high, give yourself a big pat on the back. If you've doubled your mileage since Lesson Four, don't rest and relax—go around the block one more time.

REVIEW

The food diary will continue to be one of your most valuable tools for some time. This is because it gives immediate feedback about all of your eating behaviors. The sooner after a meal you fill it out, the more effective it will be in sensitizing you to your style of eating and the content of your meals.

Consider How You Are Doing.

- Are you still keeping track with the weekly diaries?
  Yes_____ No_____

- Do you remember why you are doing these exercises one at a time—so slowly? Yes_____ No_____

- Are you continuing to do the cue elimination exercises:

	Yes	No
1. Eating in your Designated Appropriate Eating Place?	_____	_____
2. Sitting at a different place at the table?	_____	_____
3. When eating, *only* eating?	_____	_____
4. Reducing visual cues—food stored out of sight, in opaque containers, etc.?	_____	_____
5. Alternate foods?	_____	_____
6. All serving dishes off the table?	_____	_____

If not, refer back to Lesson Three, review the techniques, and try again.

If you want additional feedback, make and use a copy of the Behavior Checklist you used for the maintenance week (Lesson Six).

New behaviors are fragile and must be practiced over and over until they become habits. As we emphasized in the first lessons, weight loss without maintenance is worthless. The object of these exercises is to introduce new eating behaviors to you and have you *over*-practice until they become habits. Later in this lesson we will introduce a technique to help you keep track of your new eating behaviors and give you direct feedback on your progress and maintenance during the next few weeks.

Behavior Chains and Alternate Activities

In Lesson Seven the concept was introduced that behaviors are linked together in chains; that is, one behavior can make the immediately following behavior more or less probable. For example, buying a bag of potato chips increases the probability of a snack. In this case a behavior prior to the snack influences the probability of the snack. (If you hadn't purchased the potato chips, you wouldn't have eaten them.)

We developed this conceptual framework and demonstrated how it can be used to control food intake. The concept is quite simple. A behavior such as eating is preceded by an immediately antecedent behavior such as opening the refrigerator door. This behavior, too, has an antecedent, entering the kitchen—and so forth, back to finishing dinner an hour before and feeling full.

If your chain of behaviors is broken at any point, you will probably not continue to the final behavior in the chain—eating. The earlier you break the chain, the easier it is to unlink the chain of activities. The interventions (breaks) can be quite simple. In the example given in the last lesson, we substituted an exciting book for a dull TV show, a nap for boredom, and an alternate food for cheesecake.

Many times the behavior chain cannot be identified, or you will find yourself on the brink of the terminal behavior of eating before you are even aware of heading toward food. In this case we proposed activities that you could directly substitute for eating. These activities were of two types: things that you have to do, such as errands, washing dishes, and paying bills; and things that are enjoyable, such as hobbies, sleep, sex, taking a walk, and listening to music. We suggested you begin a substitute activity as soon as you have a craving for food.

Another strategy was simply to interpose time between you and a snack. Set a clock or cooking timer to help you interject progressively longer periods of time between the links in the behavior chain.

The assignment last week had three parts:

1. You were to write down a behavior chain, starting with eating (the terminal or final behavior in the chain) and working backwards to the beginning. You were asked to look for a weak link in the chain where you could substitute an alternate activity. The earlier in the chain you make this substitution, the easier it is to break the chain.
2. You were to write down at least three necessary and three pleasant activities that could be substituted for eating in a behavioral chain.

3. Finally, you were to substitute an activity from your list for a link in the chain, or for an inappropriate eating episode or snack.

Does This Discussion of Behavior Chains Make Sense to You?

- The theory of behavior chains? (page 120)
- Alternate activities, their definition or use? (page 121)
- Why or how to substitute alternate activities for antecedent events to disrupt behavior chains? (page 139)
- What were some of the occasions where you made a successful substitution?

  1. ______________________________

  2. ______________________________

- Were there some additional substitutions you could have made?

  1. ______________________________

  2. ______________________________

These techniques can be very useful if they are systematically applied to your inappropriate eating. Many of us are trapped into daily habit patterns that lead to extra eating—to consumption of food that we would not even be tempted by if it weren't for the circumstances that lead up to it. This technique of changing behavior patterns is the way to liberate yourself from that unnecessary eating.

NEW TOPIC: EATING BEHAVIORS—CHANGING YOUR EATING STYLE

Many people who are overweight have an eating style that leads to excess calorie consumption. Often mealtime is seen as a challenge, an effort, or something to be gotten over with as soon as possible because of its long association with gaining weight. It is partly this eating style—eating rapidly, and often excessively without knowing it—that can lead to many pounds of excess weight over the years.

Physiologically, if you eat rapidly, there isn't time for your brain to sense that your body has been fed and to turn off your hunger. There isn't time for the food to be partially digested in the stomach, and the stomach and intestines in turn to release the necessary hormones to send the proper signals to the brain to signify satiation or fullness. For the rapid eater, by the time this feeling comes, you have already consumed too much. The feeling then becomes one of being stuffed. Unfortunately by then it's too late.

Many of the "new" eating behaviors that I will be introducing sound simple, but they're really extremely difficult to master—for example putting your fork down between bites. This leads to an automatic delay of food consumption. But for someone who is used to constant eating during meals, putting one's fork down between bites is a most difficult skill to master.

Chewing thoroughly and swallowing between each bite is another simple, but difficult skill that only becomes a habit over time.

Pausing in the middle of a meal, taking your time to eat, and protecting yourself at the end of meals by eliminating leftovers, are similar skills.

It is this type of eating behavior, and one additional one, that often distinguishes the chronically overweight from their thin counterparts. The other skill is learning to taste food again. And enjoy it!

It is ironic that in spite of having a more acute awareness and sensitivity to the environment of food cues, the overweight person often forgets—or is afraid of the sense of taste. Food is eaten with great haste, with very little time taken to savor it—perhaps with the unconscious feeling that the pleasure is not deserved, or that someone will find out, or that there won't be enough food, or that eating simply must be gotten over with.

In these eating behavior exercises I want you to learn to slow down, to take your time, to savor your food, and to enjoy yourself. You will find that an average meal can be stretched out for an amazingly long period of time, that a lot of flavor is packed into foods, and that you can be satisfied with much less if you take the time to enjoy it.

Try to give yourself as much of an advantage as possible. These techniques are especially difficult if you live alone, because of the boredom factor. By contrast, eating with a companion makes it easier; it has the additional enjoyment of conversation, and the diversion of being with someone helps make it a social occasion.

It's especially important to try to avoid doing unrelated things while eating—to pay full attention to the food. One of the leading distractions associated with excess weight is television. When you are occupied with other activities like watching television, your mind is not focused on the behavior of eating; your food is consumed, often automatically in a semi-hypnotic trance.

When people are asked what they've eaten after having eaten while watching an exciting television show, there is often little or no recall for either the type of food or the quantity consumed. This obviously leads to food intake limited only by the supply of food, or the capacity of the stomach to expand.

Don't feel bad if you don't master each new behavior in one day. These so-called simple behaviors are extremely difficult to learn. For example, people who habitually eat in front of a television set usually feel a sense of hunger when their mealtime program comes on. Almost like Pavlov's dogs, they begin to salivate and feel an urge to eat. This conditioned response lasts from 12 to 15 weeks even after they have completely stopped the habit of eating with their program. But eventually the TV stimulus fades and returns to neutral in terms of food. Eventually the six o'clock news is no longer a dinner gong.

Changing the Act of Eating

The behavior you will work on this week is the actual act of eating. Many people who are overweight have a habit of eating as much food as fast as possible without pause. If you compare the bites per minute of an overweight person with those of a normal-weight person, you will see that thin people eat fast at first, but soon slow down. People who are overweight tend to keep eating rapidly throughout the meal.

Eating fast, without pausing or even slowing down, is a fattening habit. It leads to excessive eating. It takes time for the food you eat to be absorbed into your system and reduce your hunger. There is a better chance of becoming satiated, of feeling full, and a much better chance of enjoying your meal, if you slow down—take thirty minutes instead of five. By slowing down your rate of eating you may find a dramatic change in how you eat, and you will feel no more hungry than when you ate more.

Telling you to eat more slowly may be helpful, but introducing specific techniques to help you eat more slowly is a better way to approach the problem. For instance, most people have the habit of placing more food on thier forks while they are still chewing the previous forkful. As soon as they swallow their food they place more food in their mouths, and refill their forks. If you can learn to swallow the food in your mouth before adding more to your fork, you will automatically extend the length of time a meal takes and allow yourself more time to enjoy food.

HOMEWORK

The long-term goal of this week's assignment is to swallow the food from each bite before any more is added to your eating utensils. The best way to do this, and change your eating pattern, is to put your utensils down after each bite, and to not pick them up until the bite has been swallowed. In the case of handheld food such as a hamburger, put the food down between bites, in the same way you would put down a fork or spoon.

Like eating in one place, if putting your utensils down after each bite is not already a habit, establishing the behavior pattern may be difficult. At first it will feel silly, awkward, and uncomfortable. And you will tend to forget to do it.

There are two ways of establishing the habit of putting utensils down between bites: first, simply to do it; secondly, work up to it gradually. If you have to take it gradually, start by observing how frequently you currently put your eating utensils down, and then try to increase the frequency. If you find that you can put your fork down once every four bites now, work toward doing it once every two bites, and eventually after each bite. If you find it hard to remember everytime, it often helps to enlist the help of an observer.

The best form of feedback on progress in this technique is with simple ratios: e.g., 1:8, 1:4, 1:1, of bites to "fork downs." Record the ratio in the last column in your Food Diary this coming week, and see if you can make the 1:1 ratio a habit. To determine what your ratio is, count your bites for five minutes, and at the same time keep track of the number of times you put your fork or spoon down. For example, 50 bites with the utensils put down ten times would be a ratio of 10:50, or 1:5.

Either do the counting yourself, or have someone with you count for you during the first five minutes of your meals. This technique is like eating in one place, or only eating while eating—it sounds simple, but can be very difficult when you try to do it.

You must plan to take some time to change your old habits and introduce new ones. Be creative in your approach. One person bought himself a new place setting of utensils. He found that if he set his place with this new knife, fork, and spoon rather than his usual ones, he automatically remembered to eat differently, to slow down, and to put the utensils down between bites. The unfamiliar feel of the new eating utensils reminded him to use his new eating habits.

Similar techniques include the use of special place mats, or anything that makes your eating place special. To help you keep track of your bite-fork ratio, it often helps to have a card that says "count," or a block or pyramid with different ratio numbers on different sides on the table with the appropriate side (showing the ratio you are striving for) turned toward you.

If you are already successfully putting your fork down after each bite, or if you have found it easy to do, jump ahead and try an additional delaying technique: Only put more food on your fork after you swallow each bite. Then introduce a two-minute delay at some point in your meal. This can be either after 3 or 4 minutes of eating, or after a specific course, like the salad. Take the two minutes to talk, to relax, and to enjoy what you have eaten.

However, if you have trouble putting down your utensils between bites, concentrate only on that. It can be a difficult eating pattern to develop, and it should be practiced exclusively until it becomes a habit.

Be creative! There are many ways to stretch out a meal. Try to use as many delaying techniques as possible. Eating should be pleasurable. You should have time to taste, to chew, to experience all of the food you eat. Practice being more of a gourmet. Relax, slow down, and enjoy your food by concentrating on its taste, texture, sight, and smell.

Do You Feel Comfortable About This New Technique?

- Do you have any questions about the reason for putting your eating utensils down between bites? Yes______ No______

- Do you understand how to do it? Yes______ No______ (page 143)

- If you already put your utensils down between bites (always), what is your next step? (Answer: Learn to swallow between bites with my utensils on the table, and then to put in a two-minute delay in mid-meal.)

The homework assignment for this week is:

A. Keep track of your extra activity and convert the minutes to calories and record your miles of walking on the Daily Activity Record.

B. Keep track of your meals, snacks, and degree of hunger and fill in your eating ratio on the Lesson Eight Food Diary. Record any additional eating-delay techniques you have used.

C. Continue to carry out the cue elimination exercises. Is your food stored out of sight?
Yes______ No______

D. Keep burning up those calories and lowering your set point.

DAILY ACTIVITY RECORD

(Fill in miles per day walked and minutes of exercise or extra activities)

	Monday		**Tuesday**		**Wednesday**		**Thursday**		**Friday**		**Saturday**		**Sunday**	
	Miles	**Calories**	**Miles**	**Calories**	**Miles**	**Calories**	**Miles**	**Calories**	**Miles**	**Calories**	**Miles**	**Calories**	**Miles**	**Calories**
Miles Walked														
Activity or Exercise	**Mins.**	**Calories**	**Mins.**	**Calories**	**Mins.**	**Calories**	**Mins.**	**Calories**	**Mins.**	**Calories**	**Mins.**	**Calories**	**Mins.**	**Calories**

Use the table on page 109 and 110 to calculate the caloric equivalent of each activity. If your activity is not included, chose one from the list that is similar.

FOOD DIARY — Lesson Eight Sample

Day of Week Monday Date

Time	Minutes Spent Eating	M/S	H	Activity While Eating	Location of Eating	Food Type and Quantity	Eating Ratio
6:00 7:20 - 7:30	10min	M	0	Paper	Kitchen	Coffee Cereal	1:8
8:15 - 8:20	5min	S	0	Talking	Work	Coffee Donut	1:8
11:00 3:30 - 3:40	10min	M	3	Reading	Restaur.	Hamburg.	1:4
4:00 6-7	1hr.	M	2	T.V.	D.R.	Beef TV Dinner Ice Cream	1:1
9:00 10:30 - 10:45	15min	S	0	T.V.	L.R.	Ice Cream	1:2

M/S: Meal or Snack; H: Degree of Hunger (0 = None, 1 = Some, 2 = Normal, 3 = Good Healthy Hunger, 4 = Ravenous)

FOOD DIARY — Lesson Eight

Day of Week ____________________ Date ____________________

Time	Minutes Spent Eating	M/S	H	Activity While Eating	Location of Eating	Food Type and Quantity	Eating Ratio
6:00							
11:00							
4:00							
9:00							

M/S: Meal or Snack; H: Degree of Hunger (0 = None, 1 = Some, 2 = Normal, 3 = Good Healthy Hunger, 4 = Ravenous)

FOOD DIARY — Lesson Eight

Day of Week ____________________ Date ____________________

Time	Minutes Spent Eating	M/S	H	Activity While Eating	Location of Eating	Food Type and Quantity	Eating Ratio
6:00							
11:00							
4:00							
9:00							

M/S: Meal or Snack; H: Degree of Hunger (0 = None, 1 = Some, 2 = Normal, 3 = Good Healthy Hunger, 4 = Ravenous)

FOOD DIARY — Lesson Eight

Day of Week ____________________ Date ____________________

Time	Minutes Spent Eating	M/S	H	Activity While Eating	Location of Eating	Food Type and Quantity	Eating Ratio
6:00							
11:00							
4:00							
9:00							

M/S: Meal or Snack; H: Degree of Hunger (0 = None, 1 = Some, 2 = Normal, 3 = Good Healthy Hunger, 4 = Ravenous)

FOOD DIARY — Lesson Eight

Day of Week ______________ Date ______________

Time	Minutes Spent Eating	M/S	H	Activity While Eating	Location of Eating	Food Type and Quantity	Eating Ratio
6:00							
11:00							
4:00							
9:00							

M/S: Meal or Snack; H: Degree of Hunger (0 = None, 1 = Some, 2 = Normal, 3 = Good Healthy Hunger, 4 = Ravenous)

FOOD DIARY — Lesson Eight

Day of Week ______________ Date ______________

Time	Minutes Spent Eating	M/S	H	Activity While Eating	Location of Eating	Food Type and Quantity	Eating Ratio
6:00							
11:00							
4:00							
9:00							

M/S: Meal or Snack; H: Degree of Hunger (0 = None, 1 = Some, 2 = Normal, 3 = Good Healthy Hunger, 4 = Ravenous)

FOOD DIARY — Lesson Eight

Day of Week ______________ Date ______________

Time	Minutes Spent Eating	M/S	H	Activity While Eating	Location of Eating	Food Type and Quantity	Eating Ratio
6:00							
11:00							
4:00							
9:00							

M/S: Meal or Snack; H: Degree of Hunger (0 = None, 1 = Some, 2 = Normal, 3 = Good Healthy Hunger, 4 = Ravenous)

FOOD DIARY — Lesson Eight

Day of Week ____________________ Date ____________________

Time	Minutes Spent Eating	M/S	H	Activity While Eating	Location of Eating	Food Type and Quantity	Eating Ratio
6:00							
11:00							
4:00							
9:00							

M/S: Meal or Snack; H: Degree of Hunger (0 = None, 1 = Some, 2 = Normal, 3 = Good Healthy Hunger, 4 = Ravenous)

LESSON NINE

PRE-PLANNING— HEADING OFF THE URGES

WEIGH-IN AND HOMEWORK

Weigh yourself and record your weight on your Personal Weight Record. Graph your weight changes and compare it with the "average" line on your weight graph.

Using the calories of extra activity and the miles walked recorded this past week on the Daily Activity Record, graph the calories and miles on the portion of the Daily Energy-Out (activity) Graph (p. 108) for Lesson Eight.

Check your homework, and give yourself credit towards your refund on your Homework Credit Sheet.

Look Over Your Homework.

- Is your Lesson Eight Food Diary complete?
  Yes______ No______

- Has the Eating Ratio column been completely filled in?
  Yes______ No______

REVIEW

Lesson Eight discussed the fact that overweight people tend to eat faster and more continuously than thin people. You were asked to interrupt this tendency by adding a behavior that forced you to eat more slowly: putting your fork down between bites. The method of observation you used was either self-report (you counted your bites and the number of times you put your utensils down), or someone else counted for you. A ratio of forkfuls to swallows was suggested as a way of keeping track of how well you adopted this new habit. Several other behaviors and awareness exercises were suggested as ways to slow down and enjoy more.

The final point of the last lesson was positive "cuing"—helpful reminders of the changes you want to make. These are not easy to establish; indeed, one of the most difficult parts of the entire program is cueing—building reminders of the assigned behaviors into your environment. But they are well worth the effort: A card on the table, a reminder from your spouse, or a block or pyramid on the table with numbers painted on it can be a very effective reminder of, say, your desired eating ratio for that meal.

How Did You Do With This Technique?

- Did you have any problems with the idea or with the mechanics of eating slowly? Yes______ No______

- Do you understand why it is a useful technique? Yes______ No______ (page 140)

- My eating ratio today was______ : ______.

Eating slowly is an important habit to keep practicing. For the next few weeks continue eating slowly and continue to record an eating ratio in the last column of the food diary.

For those who had mastered putting their utensils down after each bite, we suggested additional techniques—that they swallow food between bites and put a time delay of two minutes into the meal, either at a pre-set time or after a certain course (like salad). During this time you were instructed simply to sit and talk, think pleasant thoughts, listen to the radio, or leave the table and do some alternate activity. This delay will allow time to pass, and the time will enable your brain to sense that your stomach has been fed.

Has This Been Effective?

- Did you try any of these techniques? Yes______ No______

  Which ones?____________________________________

  ____

- Did you see how they can be useful techniques? Yes______ No______ (page 141)

Remember, the more time you spend not eating, the less you will consume.

NEW TECHNIQUE: PRE-PLANNING WHAT YOU EAT

Pre-planning is a technique many people find very useful in controlling their food intake. Unfortunately, it is a technique that almost everyone finds correspondingly difficult. Pre-planning is an unusual way of thinking about food and the circumstances of eating. It is a technique designed to minimize the number of last-minute decisions about what to eat, and to diminish the effect of sudden impulses to eat. It is a very effective way to deal with high-calorie foods before they reach your plate.

Pre-planning can become a very strong habit and can be especially useful when you are going to a party or out to eat at a restaurant. By thinking ahead you can plan strategies for these situations. If your strategies are thought out in advance, you will have a greater tendency to limit your intake than if you had not planned at all. Thinking ahead relieves you of the necessity for on-the-spot decisions.

When you pre-plan, you pre-decide when and what to eat. For example, you might decide that after a 10:00 a.m. snack of coffee and a banana you will not have anything else to eat until 12:30, when you have scheduled a bran muffin and a diet cola. If someone offers you a doughnut at 11:00, you will be more likely to turn it down if you have planned in advance not to eat at that time. This is especially true when your meals and snacks are committed to a written schedule. If that extra doughnut isn't on the plan, it is less tempting.

Another example would be pre-planning for dinner at a good restaurant. You would think ahead about the dinner, so you would know what you were going to eat when you got there. If you plan for one cocktail, a fish entree with a green salad (dressing on the side), and sherbet, you stand a better chance of not going along with the crowd and having three cocktails, soup, Beef Wellington, and chocolate souffle.

If you enter the restaurant with a strategy, with preferences thought out in advance, you will be less influenced by impulse, and less tempted by high-calorie foods. When the second round of cocktails starts, you will still be working on your first one. When that extravagantly tempting menu is passed to you, you will be set to look at the fish section, and when dessert is proposed, you will be ready to order sherbet.

Because pre-planning involves a fundamental change in the way you think about food and social situations, the technique should be approached slowly, a step at a time. At first you should plan only one meal or snack a day. When you are able to pre-plan one meal and consistently follow the plan, increase your planning by one additional meal or snack a day. Keep increasing the amount of pre-planning until you are able to predict most of the food you will eat every day.

The object of this exercise is to develop the skill of anticipating all of your eating behaviors in advance, and being able to pre-plan all of the food you eat. With the proper use of this technique, impulse eating will disappear.

The technique of pre-planning is divided into four parts. It is a set of activities that will develop into habit patterns over a long period of time if you conscientiously practice every day.

As has been emphasized with all of the techniques in this book, you should not feel like you are in a race. Everyone develops the ability to pre-plan at a different rate. If you start feeling bad about the technique, or guilty because you are not able to do it completely, then you may be trying too hard. You should pre-plan fewer meals, and maintain that number until it feels comfortable to increase again.

These are the steps:

1. Set aside a time each day to think ahead and plan your food intake for at least part of that day. The goal will be to include in your planning all food (and drink) that has significant caloric value.
2. Write down on your food diary the time, place, type of food, and amount of food you think you will eat during the day—make a menu. But be realistic about the amount of pre-planning you start with. Don't expect to pre-plan three meals a day until you have tried to pre-plan one meal a day.

   When you write down your pre-planned meal or meals on your food diary, use a pen or pencil of a different color than the one you are accustomed to using. Later, after you have eaten your pre-planned meal, take out your regular pen and check your predictions. Correct your pre-planned menu with your regular pen. As you become a better pre-planner, the number of two-colored entries will decrease. Wait until you are consistently successful in pre-planning one meal a day before you increase to two meals a day.
3. Try to *plan ahead* for eating out and for parties. Develop pre-planned strategies: How many drinks will I have? What would really taste good besides Steak Diane? If I cannot avoid a high-calorie entree, can I eat only part of it, and eat that portion over a longer period of time?
4. If you find it hard to stick to pre-planning meals or snacks, one

helpful technique is to partially *prepare your food* in the morning, label it for the time of consumption, and put it in a special place. When the time comes to snack or eat, it is ready. The tendency to go on and eat more, or to eat at the wrong time is minimized.

Is This All Clear to You?

- Do you understand the concept of pre-planning? Yes______ No______ (page 157)

- Do you understand how to do the exercise, using two colored pens? Yes______ No______ (page 158)

- When are you going to pre-plan, and for which meal or snack?
  Pre-planning time:______
  Which meal or snack?______

- Do you see how pre-planning can be used for parties, and social functions?
  1. For drinks, hors d'oeuvres, and desserts.
  2. For pre-planning portion size—and leaving some behind.
  3. For learning to eat more slowly—with control.

- Do any of the pre-planning techniques not make sense?

- 1. Preparing snacks and meals in advance?
  Yes______ No______
  2. Thinking ahead about dining out or going to parties?
  Yes______ No______

SHOPPING: THE FORGOTTEN SKILL

The supermarket is a dangerous place. Like a restaurant menu, it is designed by experts to encourage the dieter (as well as other shoppers) to buy too much—to buy large quantities, to impulsively buy high-fat or calorically dense but well-displayed foods, or to select easy "convenience" foods, at too high a caloric "cost"—and consequently, to eat too much. Most of us have shopped all our lives without concern and without asking questions such as "How did this get in this location?" "Why is that item at the checkout stand?" "Why are the cookies at the end of the aisle?"

Don't be fooled. It's all designed for maximum appeal, maximum buying, and maximum sales of high-profit items. For the dieter, unfortunately this includes the calorically dense pre-prepared foods, sweets, and snack foods. The advertising strategy appeals particularly to the palate of the overweight person, with an emphasis on the combinations of sweet and fat (for example, candy and icings), and fat and salt (for example, chips). Even "health" foods like granola bars take advantage of our snacking habits—without telling us about the sugar that makes them appeal to our taste buds.

If you need help with the caloric content of foods, use the calorie counter you purchased four weeks ago—at the end of Lesson Five. Translate the calories into every day terms, like ten extra potato chips a day will mean almost one pound a month of weight gain—ten pounds a year! If you can eat those extra chips, you will have to lose—on top of your current weight—an extra ten pounds.

There are six golden rules for food shopping. They should be embedded in your mind, in your memory, and if necessary, written on the outside of your checkbook before you go to the supermarket:

1. *Eat before you go.* Many studies have shown that the purchasing of high-calorie "junk food" is markedly increased when a shopper is hungry. If you shop after a meal, you will buy fewer fattening and fewer impulse food items. If it's not in the house, the chances are you won't leave home to get it.
2. *Make a list.* Supermarkets sell more if they can appeal to your impulsiveness. If you are at the mercy of someone who can make food look good, you haven't got a fighting chance. If you have a list of what you need for the following week, or what you need for a specific meal, you can go through the market more easily. Keep telling yourself, I'm here to buy X, Y, Z, not Twinkies, Donuts and Danish.
3. *Preplan.* This is very important. Before you walk in those doors, commit yourself to your fundamental purpose: To replenish the pantry. The lady passing out samples, the yummies at the checkout stand, that extra special display of cookies, the sale of ice cream bars you didn't know about—ignore them all. Plan to walk through, purchase the items on your list, and walk out.
4. *Stick to the periphery.* It is here that you will find vegetables and fruits—foods that you prepare yourself—and foods that allow you to control the amount of added fat.
5. *Purchase un-prepared foods.* You will have a better chance of excluding extra fat and salt—and also you can augment taste more easily with herbs and spices—they can bring some of the fun back to eating.

6. *Don't take extra cash.* Not only will it burn a hole in your pocket, it will make a bump in your belly.

When you go to the supermarket, or the convenience store, you're entering hostile territory. Be prepared, and you won't get hurt.

HOMEWORK

Turn now to the Daily Behavior Checklist for this week. You will see that pre-planning is the principal homework assignment provided for. Each day indicate whether you did pre-plan a meal and how successful you were. Adapt the scoring system as follows: If you *tried* (but were unsuccessful) rate yourself "1." If you got so far as to write your diary in two colors, rate yourself "2." If you actually were able to *pre-plan accurately* at least *75 percent* of the time, rate yourself "3." Estimate your degree of success by how much of the pre-planned meal had to be corrected with another color ink after you ate the meal.

This is a difficult assignment. It takes time to pre-plan, and time is very hard to come by. Being able to pre-plan is a matter of establishing priorities. If this technique takes too much away from the rest of your life or interferes with your lifestyle, it may be necessary to approach it very gradually. If you do master it, you will find that pre-planning is one of the most powerful techniques for helping you limit your food intake.

Many people find that pre-planning changes their entire outlook on food. There is no longer uncertainty about what they will eat or fear of going out of control. When all of your intake is pre-planned, there is no longer a temptation to snack. It is a very useful tool for decreasing total caloric intake and gaining a feeling of greater control over your eating behaviors.

The homework assignment for this week is:

A. Shopper's Helper to be reviewed before every shopping trip for food.

B. Daily Behavior Checklist.

C. Daily Activity Record

D. Food Diary (preplanning worksheet)

SHOPPER'S HELPER—TO BE REVIEWED BEFORE SHOPPING

1. I have eaten—I am not hungry.
2. I have my shopping list.
3. I have pre-planned my meals.
4. I will shop the periphery.
5. I will not purchase "convenience" food.
6. I don't have extra money with me to "blow" on an unnecessary snack.

(You might write this on your checkbook—put a copy on the dashboard of the car, on the kitchen and refrigerator doors—or anywhere else *in sight*, so you will review it over and over.)

DAILY BEHAVIOR CHECKLIST — Lesson Nine

Points: Most of the time = 3
Sometimes = 2
Tried but did not succeed = 1

	Mon	Tue	Wed	Thu	Fri	Sat	Sun
Preplanned a: Breakfast							
Lunch							
Dinner							
Snack							
Corrected my plan after eating							
Took my shopper's helper to the market, and reviewed it before shopping							

DAILY ACTIVITY RECORD

(Fill in miles per day walked and minutes of exercise or extra activities)

	Monday		Tuesday		Wednesday		Thursday		Friday		Saturday		Sunday	
	Miles	Calories	Miles	Calories	Miles	Calories	Miles	Calories	Miles	Calories	Miles	Calories	Miles	Calories
Miles Walked														
Activity or Exercise	Mins.	Calories	Mins.	Calories	Mins.	Calories	Mins.	Calories	Mins.	Calories	Mins.	Calories	Mins.	Calories

Use the table on page 109 and 110 to calculate the caloric equivalent of each activity. If your activity is not included, chose one from the list that is similar.

FOOD DIARY — Lesson Nine
(Preplanning Worksheet)

Sample

Day of Week Monday Date ______

Time	M/S	Location of Eating	Food Type and Quantity: Planned	Food Type and Quantity: Actual (If Different)
6:00				
7:00	M	Brk. Rm	1 Bowl Cereal 1 c. coffee	
10:00	S	Kitchen	1 c. Coffee	1 donut
11:00				
12:00	M	Brk. Rm	1 Chick. Sand. 1 gl. Ice Tea	2 cookies
3:00	S	Kitchen	1 gl. milk	
4:00				
6:00	M	Kitchen	Beef TV Dinner 1 gl. milk	
9:00				
10:15	S	TV Room		1 Beer

M/S: Meal or Snack
Correct your plan in different colored ink.

FOOD DIARY — Lesson Nine
(Preplanning Worksheet)

Day of Week ____________________ Date ____________________

Time	M/S	Location of Eating	Food Type and Quantity: Planned	Food Type and Quantity: Actual (If Different)
6:00				
11:00				
4:00				
9:00				

M/S: Meal or Snack
Correct your plan in different colored ink.

FOOD DIARY — Lesson Nine
(Preplanning Worksheet)

Day of Week ____________________ Date ____________________

			Food Type and Quantity	
Time	M/S	Location of Eating	Planned	Actual (If Different)
6:00				
11:00				
4:00				
9:00				

M/S: Meal or Snack
Correct your plan in different colored ink.

FOOD DIARY — Lesson Nine
(Preplanning Worksheet)

Day of Week ____________________ Date ____________________

			Food Type and Quantity	
Time	M/S	Location of Eating	Planned	Actual (If Different)
6:00				
11:00				
4:00				
9:00				

M/S: Meal or Snack
Correct your plan in different colored ink.

FOOD DIARY — Lesson Nine
(Preplanning Worksheet)

Day of Week ____________________ Date ____________________

			Food Type and Quantity	
Time	M/S	Location of Eating	Planned	Actual (If Different)
6:00				
11:00				
4:00				
9:00				

M/S: Meal or Snack
Correct your plan in different colored ink.

FOOD DIARY — Lesson Nine
(Preplanning Worksheet)

Day of Week ____________________ Date ____________________

			Food Type and Quantity	
Time	M/S	Location of Eating	Planned	Actual (If Different)
6:00				
11:00				
4:00				
9:00				

M/S: Meal or Snack
Correct your plan in different colored ink.

FOOD DIARY — Lesson Nine
(Preplanning Worksheet)

Day of Week ____________________ Date ____________________

			Food Type and Quantity	
Time	M/S	Location of Eating	Planned	Actual (If Different)
6:00				
11:00				
4:00				
9:00				

M/S: Meal or Snack
Correct your plan in different colored ink.

FOOD DIARY — Lesson Nine
(Preplanning Worksheet)

Day of Week ____________________ Date ____________________

			Food Type and Quantity	
Time	M/S	Location of Eating	Planned	Actual (If Different)
6:00				
11:00				
4:00				
9:00				

M/S: Meal or Snack
Correct your plan in different colored ink.

LESSON TEN

CUE ELIMINATION, PART TWO— SWITCHING MORE SIGNALS

WEIGH-IN AND HOMEWORK

Weigh yourself and graph your weight change.

Check your homework.

- Is your Lesson Nine Behavior Checklist complete?
  Yes______ No______
- Have you become comfortable with pre-planning?
  Yes______ No______
- Did you take your Shopper's Helper to the market this week?
  Yes______ No______
- Did you write it on your checkbook for easy reference?
  Yes______ No______
- Are you taking time to identify other eating problems?
  Yes______ No______

Give yourself credit for your homework.

Plot the calories of extra activity, and the miles on your pedometer for the past week on your Daily Energy-Out (activity) Graph (p. 108).

REVIEW

Pre-planning

The technique of pre-planning was introduced last week. A good way to increase the probability that your behavior will be different in the future is to make definite plans and commit yourself to a course of action in advance. You will be more likely to limit your food intake if you plan ahead to eat specific foods at pre-selected times and places. It's much more effective than simply saying to yourself, "I'm going to be more careful about what I eat."

Self-instruction and expectation play a large part in how hungry you are during the day. If each meal and snack is scheduled, and you stick to the schedule long enough, the question of whether or not you are hungry will not cross your mind when food is not on your schedule—for example, when candy is served unexpectedly at the office, or when you pass a vending machine or a bakery. Regardless of the feeling, you won't eat because you haven't planned for it; and the strength of the stimulus telling you to eat will be weakened each time you ignore it.

Pre-planning is a time-consuming project at first. Like the Food Diary, it takes much less time after you've practiced doing it. In fact, the time used thinking about filling it out may be the most time-consuming and anxiety-provoking part of this technique.

Pre-planning can be approached in steps. Pre-plan one meal a day, then add a second meal, or a snack, and continue until the whole day's food intake is planned in advance. For some people, for example those who plan meals for a family, this technique will be easy. For others it may take a month or more before the ability to plan each meal in advance becomes a habit.

Pre-planning can be divided into a series of steps: First, designate a time each day to think ahead and plan meals and snacks, at first only one meal or snack for each day. Second, actually write down these plans on your Food Diary. Third, correct your pre-planned meals with a different colored pen after you eat a meal.

These different colored notations emphasize the difference between the amount and type of food you planned and food you actually ate. If snacks are difficult to plan, it might be easier to prepare them in advance, label them for a specific time, and eat them when you planned to snack.

Another use of pre-planning is at parties or when you go out to dinner. If you anticipate an unavoidable large meal, you can plan to decrease your food intake earlier in the day to make up for a planned calorie excess. You can also plan strategies for parties: how many drinks you will have, how many hors d'oeuvres, how much cake you will have for dessert.

How Did This Go?

- Do you have any questions about the theory, definition, or reason for pre-planning? Yes______ No______ (page 157)

- Do you have any questions about how the pre-planning should be done? Yes______ No______ (page 158)

- Were you able to pre-plan a restaurant meal and actually carry out your contingency plan? Yes______ No______

- Did you notice any changes in your eating pattern, particularly with respect to impulse eating?
  Yes______ No______

It is all right to switch equal foods like peas and beans, or simply to anticipate a general type of food when you plan your eating at a restaurant. In pre-planning the spirit is more important than the letter of the theory.

The final point in pre-planning was very important: changing your food-buying behavior by pre-planning when you will shop and what you will buy. Before you shop for food, review your Shopper's Helper, and make a shopping list which includes everything you are going to buy, very specifically listed by brand name and quantity. Go to the store on a full stomach to avoid impulse buying, don't take extra money, and try not to vary from your shopping list. This will help you avoid buying snack foods and products which contain only empty calories. Food that is not bought and is not within easy reach will not be eaten.

Do You Feel You Made Progress?

- Did you go shopping on a full stomach?
  Yes______ No______

- Did you notice a change in your attraction to impulse foods at the market? Yes______ No______

- Were you able to pre-plan and shop from a list?
  Yes________ No________

CUE ELIMINATION: PART TWO (ABOUT THOSE STARVING ARMENIANS)

In the first discussions of cue elimination (Lessons Two and Three) you were told that overweight people tend to be controlled more by environmental stimuli than thin people. They tend to be more sensitive to the smell and sight of food, and places associated with food, than their thin friends.

At that time several methods of eliminating cues (or environmental reminders) that often lead to inappropriate eating were introduced. These were:

1. Eat only at a Designated Appropriate Eating Place.
2. Change your habitual eating place at the table.
3. When you are eating, only eat—no other activities.
4. Work to reduce visual food cues: remove food from all places in the house other than appropriate storage areas. Store food in opaque containers to keep it out of sight.
5. Have alternate foods available to replace high impulse or "junk" foods.
6. Do not leave serving dishes on the table.

All of these exercises helped reduce the potency of food cues in your environment. These six rules, if followed carefully, will affect almost all inappropriate eating, and will help you build a new set of responses to former food cues. For example, by now you are probably watching the 6:00 news for information instead of for permission to eat.

All of the cue elimination exercises in Lesson Three involved stimuli that were physically removed from food. Today you will receive six additional exercises that will help you eliminate cues more closely associated with the act of eating.

These exercises appear deceptively simple, but you may find that you are not able to do all of them immediately. The more of them you can master, the higher the probability of your success in losing weight. Some of the techniques may not be applicable at all times; for example, using smaller plates when you are at a restaurant. However, most people are able to use these cue elimination techniques most of the time without difficulty.

The new exercises are as follows:

1. *Smaller Plates.* Research has shown that the size of the plate your food is served on has a large influence on how you perceive the amount of food you are eating, and consequently, how full you feel after the meal. Even though you know that the size of the plate does not make any difference—a spoonful of potatoes is basically a spoonful of potatoes—it seems like more food when it is served on a smaller plate.

   A psychology experiment demonstrated that 70 percent of the people in a weight reduction program were more satisfied with less food when it was served on a salad plate than when it was served on a dinner plate. (4)

   This week I would like you to try eating from smaller plates; try to make them a part of your daily routine.

2. *Set Some Aside.* All of us have been strongly conditioned to eat everything on our plates, and to feel guilty when we leave some behind. Whether for economy, aesthetics, or because of all the starving children in Armenia, China, or elsewhere, almost everyone has been taught this lesson. Not wasting food is usually a very well learned irrational idea. The implicit belief is that if we finish our meals and eat everything on our plate, it will benefit someone else. The unfortunate corollary to this is, "If I do not finish everything on my plate, somehow I am bad."

   One could consider the history of this concept and how possibly it evolved during times of famine. But it would serve no purpose; many of us are stuck with it, whatever its origin. It is, of course, a very false economy. It leads to eating more than we need, because we feel we must finish and not leave food to be thrown away.

   The second assignment for today is to start breaking this habit, to begin to free yourself of the compulsion to eat everything you are served. To accomplish this, leave food behind at each meal. Start out slowly: one pea, a spoonful of potatoes, or a crust of bread from your sandwich.

   It may be necessary to set the leftover food aside at the start of the meal and cover it with plastic wrap so you won't forget to leave it behind. Or, at the end of the meal, you may find it necessary to put the leftover food in the garbage immediately, to prevent yourself from eating it. (This technique can be used later for eliminating problem foods and reducing portion size.) For today, concentrate on leaving some food on your plate after every meal.

3. *Seconds*. For those eating large portions, expecially at dinner, divide the food you would normally serve yourself into two helpings, and go back for seconds when you finish the first half. This introduces a delay, and hopefully a thinking step in the middle of the meal, e.g., "Do I really want seconds or thirds?" It has the added advantage of keeping the second half of the meal warm and more enjoyable when you do eat it. Don't forget to leave some of each portion behind.
4. *Throw Away*. Throw away any food left on your plate immediately after the meal. Put scraps down the disposal, in the garbage can, or feed them to the cat. In this way they won't linger around to be nibbled on later in the evening or the next afternoon. If you do keep something, like a chicken wing or a serving of peas, pre-plan it into part of lunch or a snack for the next day. Put it in an opaque container and label it with its specific pre-planned use, for example, "John's Lunch." Don't let food hang around the house loose and uncommitted! It will reach out and tempt you to eat.
5. *Ask for Food*. Never accept food from another person unless you ask for it. Make each encounter with food a voluntary one. In restaurants, take the initiative—ask the server not to bring butter, or to take away the bread. If it is not on the table, you won't nibble on it while you wait for your meal.
6. *Minimize Contact*. Try to arrange your food contacts in ways that minimize the chances for impulse eating. For example, when you fix yourself a sandwich for lunch, put away the bread, butter, and jelly, and clean up the mess before you eat your sandwich. This will greatly reduce the likelihood that you will make a second sandwich. Food out of sight is often food out of mind.

Do You Understand the Need for This Second Set of Cue Elimination Exercises?

These exercises deal with cues or stimuli inherent in the act of eating—the previous elimination exercises dealt with more general environmental cues. Every time you sit down to eat, think of the starving Armenians and follow these six steps: (1) use small plates, (2) leave some food behind, (3) split large meals into several portions, (4) throw leftovers away or pre-plan them for a specific use, (5) ask for food when you want it, and (6) organize your environment to minimize chances for impulse eating.

CUE ELIMINATION, PART TWO

The old cue elimination exercises are still valid. The less conspicuous food is, the less you respond to environmental stimuli that remind you to eat, the better your habits will become, and the better the odds that your weight loss will be permanent.

MAINTENANCE AND THE BEHAVIOR CHECKLIST

The behavior therapies emphasize maintenance of behaviors once they have been established. The Daily Behavior Checklist is a tool to help improve the odds of successful maintenance. For the next four weeks fill in the checklist every day, and try to improve your score as the weeks progress.

When you are confident that your new eating skills are habitual, the checklist can be eliminated. On the other hand, when you feel a need to brush up on your new habits, reintroduce the checklist for a few weeks (if necessary, making additional copies for yourself). Periodic practice is one way to assure successful maintenance. In the final lesson, you will have a Maintenance Behavior Checklist.

The homework assignment for this week is:

A. Daily Behavior Checklist

B. Food Diary to continue preplanning

C. Daily Energy-Out (activity) Graph

DAILY BEHAVIOR CHECKLIST — Lesson Ten

(Answer yes or no)

	M	Tu	W	Th	F	Sa	Su
Preplanned at least one meal							
Kept up a high activity level							
Exercised at least 20 minutes							
Cue Elimination:							
smaller plates							
set some aside							
smaller seconds							
designated eating place							
throw away leftovers							
ask for food							
food contract minimized							
Still doing the "old" cue elimination exercises (Lesson 3)							

FOOD DIARY — Lesson Ten
(Preplanning Worksheet)

Day of Week ____________________ Date ____________________

			Food Type and Quantity	
Time	M/S	Location of Eating	Planned	Actual (If Different)
6:00				
11:00				
4:00				
9:00				

M/S: Meal or Snack
Correct your plan in different colored ink.

FOOD DIARY — Lesson Ten
(Preplanning Worksheet)

Day of Week ____________________ Date ____________________

			Food Type and Quantity	
Time	M/S	Location of Eating	Planned	Actual (If Different)
6:00				
11:00				
4:00				
9:00				

M/S: Meal or Snack
Correct your plan in different colored ink.

FOOD DIARY — Lesson Ten
(Preplanning Worksheet)

Day of Week ________________ Date ________________

			Food Type and Quantity	
Time	M/S	Location of Eating	Planned	Actual (If Different)
6:00				
11:00				
4:00				
9:00				

M/S: Meal or Snack
Correct your plan in different colored ink.

FOOD DIARY — Lesson Ten
(Preplanning Worksheet)

Day of Week ________________ Date ________________

			Food Type and Quantity	
Time	M/S	Location of Eating	Planned	Actual (If Different)
6:00				
11:00				
4:00				
9:00				

M/S: Meal or Snack
Correct your plan in different colored ink.

FOOD DIARY — Lesson Ten
(Preplanning Worksheet)

Day of Week ____________________ Date ____________________

			Food Type and Quantity	
Time	M/S	Location of Eating	Planned	Actual (If Different)
6:00				
11:00				
4:00				
9:00				

M/S: Meal or Snack
Correct your plan in different colored ink.

FOOD DIARY — Lesson Ten
(Preplanning Worksheet)

Day of Week ____________________ Date ____________________

			Food Type and Quantity	
Time	M/S	Location of Eating	Planned	Actual (If Different)
6:00				
11:00				
4:00				
9:00				

M/S: Meal or Snack
Correct your plan in different colored ink.

FOOD DIARY — Lesson Ten
(Preplanning Worksheet)

Day of Week ____________________ Date ____________________

			Food Type and Quantity	
Time	M/S	Location of Eating	Planned	Actual (If Different)
6:00				
11:00				
4:00				
9:00				

M/S: Meal or Snack
Correct your plan in different colored ink.

LESSON ELEVEN

IT'S TIME TO EAT OUT— How to Do It

WEIGH-IN AND HOMEWORK

Weigh yourself, record your weight on your Personal Weight Record and graph your weight change.

Homework:

- Is your Lesson Ten homework complete?
  Yes ______ No ______
- Did you pre-plan your meals on your food diary?
  Yes ______ No ______
- Did you maintain an increased activity/exercise level?
  Yes ______ No ______
- Give yourself credit for your completed homework.

REVIEW: CUE ELIMINATION, PART TWO

Last lesson's cue elimination exercises were designed to change your response to cues common in eating and food-related activities. In many ways these are harder cues to ignore than more remote environmental stimuli like television and vending machines. Food-related cues are present every time you sit down to eat.

The use of smaller plates has been found by many to be very effective in eliminating the strong cues related to meal size; smaller plates take advantage of a tendency everyone has to judge the size of a meal by how well it fills the plate.

You were asked to stop feeding the starving Armenian inside yourself and to leave some food on your plate after each meal. The effect of this exercise is to eliminate the feeling that a meal ends when the plate is clean. Unfortunately, most of us were taught this habit as children, and find it is surprisingly difficult to break.

Splitting large portions in half and going back for the second half is a way of introducing both a delay and a thinking break into the meal. By the time you decide to have the second part of the meal, you may no longer want it.

Throwing away excess food, or labeling it for its future use, eliminates the cue to eat that is usually associated with leftovers. This technique can provide an easy way of freeing yourself from an old snacking habit.

The final two cue elimination techniques were: never accept food from others—always ask for what you want, whether it is at home or in a restaurant; and minimize contact with food—the easiest way to do this is to clean up the mess you make preparing food before you eat what you have prepared. (In the process of getting all the food out again you will think twice about that second sandwich or third piece of toast and jam in the morning.)

Was Last Week's Lesson Easy or Difficult?

- Do you have any questions about last week's cue elimination exercise? Yes ______ No ______

- Did you try smaller plates? Yes ______ No ______

- Were you able to leave food behind on your plate? Yes ______ No ______

- Did it reduce the feeling that you should clean up your plate? Yes ______ No ______ (It will vanish with time.)

- Were you able to deal successfully with leftovers—either throwing them away immediately, feeding them to the cat or disposal, or pre-planning and labeling them for a specific use? Yes ______ No ______

- Did you remember to ask for food rather than blindly accept it from others? Yes ______ No ______

- Is all the food in your house out of sight?
  Yes ______ No ______

Leaving food behind can control the size of a meal, at home or at a party—when they pass the hors d'oeuvres, only eat half of one, leave some of your drink in the glass, etc. Each of the cue elimination techniques can be used in a variety of eating situations.

Two weeks ago you learned to pre-plan for a variety of situations. This included planning your food for the day, and seeing if you could stick to your plan. I had you write down your intake in advance on the Food Diary and go back and correct it at the end of the day. This one technique acts as a very potent motivator for changing eating behaviors. It leads to a marked decrease in the amount of food you eat. It eliminates spontaneity, and at the same time snacking.

I also emphasized the need for shopping skills, so that you aren't at the mercy of the merchandiser. The supermarket is ***hostile territory***. It is carefully arranged to maximize your purchase of pre-prepared high-calorie foods. These have the highest profit margin. Vegetables and unprepared foods have a much lower "value" to the market, so they are sold off to one side (on the "periphery"). The six commandments of supermarket shopping were shared with you in that lesson.

Are you still using them? Do you need a refresher? If so go back to Lesson Eight and review. If you don't buy high-calorie foods, there won't be any in the house for a midnight snack. If you don't snack, you will stand a good chance of losing and controlling your weight.

RESTAURANT EATING

By now, you're craving a meal away from the confines of home. Restaurants are a prime site for losing *"it"* (but not for losing weight) when you're on a diet. The restaurateur doesn't give you a fair chance! It's in his best interests to make the food as attractive and palatable as possible, and to design an environment that is as luxurious as possible, to help "lead you astray."

Unfortunately this often means sauces, fats, and salt. Menus are written with an eye to psychology, to urge you to go for the best (also the most profitable). Not only that, but eating is often combined with a celebration like a birthday or special treat, or Friday after a hard week at work; it is (if you're near home) a chance to be away from the kids, or (if you're on business), maybe a time when you are eating alone—for the business person, restaurant survival is a must.

The first and most important principle in dealing with someone else's cooking is preplanning. Your preplanning, not theirs! Also, try not to be a passive guest—if possible, use your influence! If you can help decide which restaurant you're going to, choose the one that's known for its "light cuisine," a salad bar, or fish. So far, so good!

But choosing the restaurant isn't the end of the battle. Think ahead about the entire occasion—at restaurants, and also at parties, and even at Aunt Minnie's Thanksgiving Dinner—whenever and wherever someone else does the cooking.

Rehearse the entire occasion in your mind. Preplan what you will do when you see a menu. What will you say when the hors d'oeuvres and drinks are served? What will you choose—and will you have to justify yourself? (NO!)

Remember you are not obligated to choose anything. What will you drink? Remember that alcohol not only contains calories (one beer = 150 calories, 1½ oz. whisky = 105 calories), it also lowers your willpower to make wise food choices, and may enhance your appetite. Sparkling water is often a good alternative; it has none of the shortcomings, yet it satisfies most of the social needs.

Even when faced with unfamiliar foods in a restaurant, some things reliably have fewer (or extra) calories. Fish, for example, can nearly always be obtained broiled or poached, and sauces can always be ordered on the side. Don't be afraid to ask the waiter not to bring the bread, or to take it back if it has been delivered. There's nothing more tempting, and nothing easier to eat by "accident" during a conversation than a piece of freshly buttered bread, while you're waiting for the entree to arrive.

Choose clear soups, rather than creamed soups. Eat (very) slowly, and leave some behind. It doesn't matter if it's mashed potatoes, peas, or filet mignon. Leave some behind, and don't take it home.

Make your decision about dessert in advance. You needn't abstain, but informed consent always helps. If you're going to have the chocolate mousse, split it with a friend, or (if you can't avoid a full serving) assure yourself ahead of time that one bite will be enough, that you'll savor it, stretch it out, and leave the rest behind. Have some idea about calories (that mousse is worth at least 300 calories per serving).

Calorie banking is another important principle to remember. If you preplan, and decide ahead of time to splurge, make up for it in advance. Save a few calories here and there so that the average over three days doesn't exceed your dietary guidelines. On the other hand—don't starve before you go out. If you do, you are a sitting duck for the menu writer—it is like going shopping on an empty stomach—you won't be able to control your appetite!

Above all, remember to preplan. Know what you're ordering, and stand up for yourself against unwanted food when you eat out. With these simple guidelines, and some practice with the menus, you won't have any trouble.

Look at the menus—with calories (pages 194 and 195) from Wendy's and McDonald's. How many calories in a Big Mac with cheese? ______ In a green salad? ______ In a chocolate milk shake? ______ In a simple hamburger? ______ In those french fries? ______ In a glass of soda water? ______ If you were going to one of these restaurants, how would you pre-plan your dinner? How well do you do with fancy foods?

HOMEWORK

This lesson's homework is an exercise in eating out. Choose a restaurant to visit. If possible, obtain a copy of the menu in advance. If it's a fancy restaurant, often the menus are posted outside. Sneak over, copy it down, and bring it home. Or, more assertively, ask the restaurant for a copy. If you can't obtain one, make up one similar to what you think you will find at the restaurant.

In the calm of your own home, look at your menu. Strip away the fancy words, and look at it in terms of the food alone. What about that entree? What's in it? If you don't know—look it up in *The Joy of Cooking* or your favorite cookbook. How many calories do you think it has? (______) (Put in calories) What about that Whopper with cheese from Burger King? (______) What about a milk shake? (______) What about an 8-oz. filet mignon? (______) What about bean burrito? (______) What about 4 oz. of chocolate mousse? (______)

Look at the menu and plan ahead. How can you negotiate your way through a dinner at the restaurant with a minimum of calories?

For hors d'oeuvres, what are the choices? How about raw vegetables? What will you say to the waiter when he brings the bread to the table? ("Please don't bring bread to my table.") What will you choose to drink? (Perrier with a twist of lemon/lime or diet soda.) What about a main course? (Broiled or poached fish would be lowest in calories—"sauces on the side please"). For soup, one that is clear, and vegetables that are simple and steamed. Desserts optional.

Write down what you're going to choose, at least by category. Get up your courage and go for it.

After your dinner out, come home and write down how well you did compared with what you had planned to do. Compare this with what would have happened if you had walked into the restaurant unprepared.

FAST FOOD MENUS

BURGER KING

Whooper	630
Whooper Jr.	370
Double Beef Whooper	850
Whooper with cheese	740
Whooper Jr. w/cheese	420
Cheeseburger	305
Fries	210
Onion Rings	270
Vanilla Shake	340
Chocolate Shake	340
Coke (12 oz.)	144
Prepackaged Salads:	
Chef Salad	180
Garden Salad	110
Pasta Salad	250
Shrimp Salad	90
Side Salad	20
Dressings (per serving):	
Blue Cheese	300
French	280
House	260
Reduced Low-Cal Italian	30
1000 Island	240

KENTUCKY FRIED CHICKEN

2-Piece dinner, drum and thigh (includes 2 pieces of chicken, mashed potato & gravy, cole slaw & roll)

Original Recipe	643
Extra Crispy	855

MCDONALDS

Hamburger	255
Cheeseburger	307
Quarter Pounder	424
Quarter Pounder with cheese	524
Big Mac	563
Fillet of Fish	432
French fries	220
Chocolate Shake	383
Vanilla Shake	352
Hot fudge Sundae	310
Egg McMuffin	327
Hot Cakes with butter and syrup	500
Scrambled Eggs	180
Sausage	206
Salads:	
Chef Salad	236
Chicken Salad	
Oriental	146
Garden Salad	91
Shrimp Salad	99
Side Salad	48
Dressings (per packet):	
Blue Cheese	342
French	228
House	326
Low Cal Vinegarette	50
Oriental	103
1000 Island	396

TACO BELL

Taco	186
Tostada	179
Bean Burrito	343
Burrito Supreme	457
Enchirito	454
Pinto 'n Cheese	168
Beefy Tostada	291

PIZZA HUT

1/2 Small 10 inch Pizza

Thin and Crispy	
Beef	490
Cheese	450
Pepperoni	430
Supreme	510
Thick and Chewy	
Beef	620
Cheese	560
Pepperoni	560
Supreme	640

WENDY'S

Single Hamburger	470
Double Hamburger	670
Triple Hamburger	850
Single with Cheese	580
Double with Cheese	800
Triple with Cheese	1040
Taco Salad	460
Chili	230
French Fries	330
Frosty	390

(lettuce, tomato, onion, pickle, mustard and catsup included on all burgers.)

DAIRY QUEEN

Small Cone	110
Small Malt	340
Small Sundae	170
Mr. Misty Freeze	500

STEAK HOUSE MENU

Appetizers

Salad Bar	75
Dressings:	
Bleu Cheese	426
French	342
1000 Island	420

Entrees

Steak - 8oz.	801
Steak - 16 oz.	1600
Fish (light color, flounder)	180
Fish (dark color, sword)	371
Chicken	598
King Crab Legs	211
Lobster Tail, medium	206

Side Dishes

Artichoke	44
Mayonnaise	99
Butter	65
Mushrooms, sautéed	150
Baked Potato with sour cream	145
Bread - 2 oz. slice	146

P.S. How many miles did you walk today? (______) How many minutes did you spend in extra activity? (______)

The homework assignment for this week is:

A. Write out a menu for a mythical restaurant ("Chez Moi")—choosing one with the lowest number of calories possible for breakfast, lunch and dinner. Make it a menu you would like to find. Now, go see how close you can come to finding a restaurant that has your ideal "dream" menu.

B. Keep track of your activity this week, and compare the miles walked and minutes of extra activity with those recorded on the Daily Activity Record for your Lesson Four homework (p. 85).

Lesson Eleven

SAMPLE MENU
("Chez Moi")

	Calories	Your Selection (Select One)	Calories
Appetizers			
______	______	______	______
______	______	______	______
______	______	______	______
______	______	______	______
Entrees			
______	______	______	______
______	______	______	______
______	______	______	______
______	______	______	______
Desserts			
______	______	______	______
______	______	______	______
______	______	______	______
______	______	______	______
Beverages			
______	______	______	______
______	______	______	______
______	______	______	______
______	______	______	______

TOTAL ______

DAILY ACTIVITY RECORD

(Fill in miles per day walked and minutes of exercise or extra activities)

	Monday		Tuesday		Wednesday		Thursday		Friday		Saturday		Sunday	
	Miles	Calories	Miles	Calories	Miles	Calories	Miles	Calories	Miles	Calories	Miles	Calories	Miles	Calories
Miles Walked														
Activity or Exercise	Mins.	Calories	Mins.	Calories	Mins.	Calories	Mins.	Calories	Mins.	Calories	Mins.	Calories	Mins.	Calories

Use the table on page 109 and 110 to calculate the caloric equivalent of each activity. If your activity is not included, chose one from the list that is similar.

LESSON TWELVE MAINTENANCE WEEK— YOU DESERVE IT

WEIGH-IN AND HOMEWORK

Weigh yourself, record your weight on your Personal Weight Record, and graph your weight change.

- Did you complete your own "dream" menu?
  Yes_______ No_______
- Did you find a restaurant that offered the type of food you used for your menu?
  Yes_______ No_______
- Did this assignment help you identify the type of restaurant where you can enjoy the food without blowing your weight control program?
  Yes_______ No_______

Give yourself credit for your completed homework

REVIEW

During the past 5 weeks you've learned a wide variety of skills to help you cope with excess eating. Beginning after the last maintenance week, you first looked at the behavior chains which have led to your habitual overeating. Many of these were identified, and you worked out programs for eliminating these habitual and unnecessary associations with food. You also changed the way you ate, your eating speed, how many times you chew each bite, and how you handle your utensils at the dinner table.

All of these techniques were designed to slow down overactive eating, and to get you back in touch with the taste and sensual nature of food. The more you can enjoy food, the less of it you will need.

Preplanning was presented in several contexts. I talked about how it is necessary to preplan each meal, to preplan the day, and especially to preplan your shopping so that Twinkies don't wind up hidden in your bedroom closet. If they're not in the house, they won't be eaten.

A whole new set of behavioral cues were talked about. They specifically related to your eating environment. The techniques you practiced included: (1) using smaller plates, (2) setting some food aside to be discarded, (3) dividing large portions into small portions, and then making a decision as to whether or not you really want to go back for seconds, (4) throwing away food left on your plate immediately after the meal, (5) asking for food rather than accepting it when it's passed to you, and (6) minimizing food contacts.

All of these exercises can help you gain control over the food rather than allowing it to control you.

Finally, restaurant eating was addressed. Most Americans eat out frequently, and enjoy it. Unfortunately restaurants are designed to make money, and one makes money by selling food that is palatable, pleasing, and usually, fattening.

There are ways around this. But you have to use all of the skills that you've developed at home to make the restaurant a safe eating place. Among the skills you need are preplanning, and the ability to recognize the caloric density of food. If you plan ahead at a time when you have already eaten, you're not at the mercy of the restaurateur who did his preplanning when he wrote his menu.

HOMEWORK

For this maintenance period, we want you to practice all of the skills you have learned in this book. Pick out and keep a record of the ones that seem particularly difficult. Continue with your activity and exercise, and practice, practice, practice!

One danger in this program is information overload. Each of the techniques is deceptively simple, and at the same time potentially difficult to master. Going back to the example of juggling — if you get too many balls in the air, you will lose control and they will all fall down. The maintenance period allows you to practice the techniques that need more time, and master what you have already taken on, before you throw another ball into the air.

The homework assignment for this week is:

A. Go over all of the techniques presented in the course to date, and select any that you do not feel confident you have mastered.

B. Fill out the Behavior Change List each evening before going to bed. Check off the boxes for the techniques you feel you have mastered, and complete the boxes for activities/exercise where you have kept track of mileage or time.

MAINTENANCE PERIOD #2 — Lesson Twelve

Behavior Change List

(Answer yes or no)

	M	Tu	W	Th	F	Sa	Su
Activity (minutes)							
calories							
Exercise (miles)							
calories							
daily total calories							
weekly total calories							
Preplanning (number of meals & snacks)							
Shopping List (yes/no)							
Cue Elimination Techniques used: 1.							
2.							
3.							
4.							
5.							
6.							

LESSON THIRTEEN

HOW WE THINK IS HOW WE EAT—THINK BEFORE YOU BUY

WEIGH-IN AND HOMEWORK

Weigh yourself, record your weight, and graph your weight change.

- My total weight loss for the first 12 weeks is______ lbs.
- My average miles per day of walking this week has been ______.
- My average minutes of extra activity have been ______.
- Last week was the second maintenance period. The reason that this was included in the program was

  ____

  ____

  (If I don't practice what I learn, I won't incorporate it into my lifestyle. I might as well not lose weight if it's only to regain it. The only insurance I have against this is practice, practice, practice.)

- During the second maintenance period you practiced six cue elimination techniques every day. List them:

1. ____________________

2. ____________________

3. ____________________

4. ____________________

5. ____________________

6. ____________________

REVIEW

During the first 12 weeks we talked about the effect of the environment on eating. The sight of a freshly baked doughnut is like a sign offering water to a thirsty traveler in the middle of the desert. It jumps out at you, and says "eat me." Prior to that there may have been no thought of food, and particularly not a high caloric, greasy, sugary doughnut.

However, knowing this doesn't help a bit. Most food cues are more subtle, like the time of day, a well composed advertisement, the sight of someone else eating, or too large a portion of food. It takes time, and repeated use of special techniques to learn to deal with these subtle cues.

Part of the difficulty comes from outside pressure, perhaps Uncle George who has dropped in and brought a chocolate cake from Aunt Minnie because that's the thing to do—and God forbid you should turn it down or eat just a small piece. It might be that special recipe or celebration, or simply everyone else ordering a big meal and you feeling awkward not going along with the crowd.

I've rehearsed and walked you through the supermarket, and you've come out unscathed. I upped the ante and had you go through a restaurant, first on paper, and finally for real.

- What three principles have you learned about eating in the real world?

1. ____________________

2. ______________________________

3. ______________________________

(1. Preplanning. Plan ahead for exactly what you'll eat.)
(2. Informed consent. If you know what you're eating, you're much less likely to eat extra calories by mistake.)
(3. Exercise is important, no matter what happens to the act of eating.)

THOUGHTS AND FEELINGS

This chapter leaves the world of the external, the cues and stimuli that turn our eating on, and begins a discussion of the internal world of thoughts and feelings, which are equally important in determining what we eat, when, where, and how much food we consume.

The next 5 lessons will discuss feelings and self-image, our irrational beliefs about food, stress and how it affects our eating, and how we can avoid it. I'll talk about people close to us, and their effect for good or bad on our weight control program. Finally, I will go over some hints about problem solving, and how to use the many techniques that you have built upon over the last 12 weeks.

- Do you agree that feelings, and opinions of one's self are important in a weight control program?
  Yes______ No______

Before we look at feelings *per se*, let's look at your self-image.

SELF-IMAGE

We all have an image of who and what we are—and an image of what our potential is. Much of this is based on a combination of childhood ideals, day-to-day reality, and secretive pressures and influences.

Our self-image tends to mesh with our repetitive thinking, particularly those negative thoughts that may be repeated over and over during the day—expecially during times of negative feelings. It is these feelings—this self-image—that keep us where we are. For example: "I'm fat." "I'll never change." "I'm a slob, otherwise I would be thin." "If I had any willpower, I'd be at the top of the heap, and thin to boot."

The easiest way to break the trap of a negative self-image is to allow yourself to project ahead to what you want to be, and begin to form an image in your mind of the new thin person that you want to become. You might not be able to achieve it all—I don't expect you to. I only want you to get the ball rolling, and to get you pointed in the right psychological direction.

Before you look at the specific attributes of your self- image, answer the questions below:

1. Can I accept the consequences of being thin?
   Yes______ No______
2. Can I face the expectations of others when I'm thin?
   Yes______ No______
3. Can I live up to my own expectations of what I will be like when I'm thin?
   Yes______ No______
4. Have I been hiding behind my weight, frightened of life, of sexuality, or of mobility and freedom?
   Yes______ No______

To help you get in touch with your thin self, I want you to write down some of the characteristics of the thin person inside you. What type of clothes will you wear? How will your day-to-day life at work and at home be different? Will you be happier, busier—or more depressed? Let go of your fantasies and try to express what you really hope for.

The future-oriented autobiography on the following pages will help you clarify your goals in a very specific way. Take some time, when you're alone, and think about each of the questions. Try to imagine yourself at some time in the future each time you answer one of the questions. If you have a close friend in this weight control program, share your opinions with him or her. Share your future autobiography with your spouse, or loved one. The more realistic it can be for you, the more closely you'll approximate it over time. Out of this scenario, a new self-image will begin to develop.

Fill in the blanks on the Future Autobiography form—with one ground rule: "Given the best of all possible worlds, with no restraint, what will my life be like when I'm thin?"

FUTURE AUTOBIOGRAPHY

My ideal weight will be ______________________

My ideal clothing size will be ______________________

When I am at this ideal weight, I will (describe what you will look like)

____

The clothes I will wear will be (style or type) ______________________

____

My day-to-day life will be (describe what will be different)

____

Some of the things I will do differently will be ______________________

____

The sports I will engage in will be ______________________

____

My social life—dating will be ______________________

____

My sex life will be ______________________

____

My home life will change by ______________________

____

My spouse/partner and I will ______________________

____

I will cope with being more attractive or sexier by ______________________

____

I will deal with the expectations of others by

____

____

Everyone needs a positive self-image. It is a part of a feeling of personal worth. Our daily lives are shaped by our self-image: how we view ourselves and value ourselves in the world.

Your self-image can be your best friend and motivator; or it can be your worst enemy and totally defeat you, depending on your perceived strengths and weaknesses. Developing, maintaining, and rehearsing a positive self-image provides you with an inner feeling of self-acceptance and self-respect that will allow you to love yourself, to love others, and not to turn to food as a substitute for what you really need in life: intimacy, a sense of effectiveness, and meaning in your life.

One way of describing our life is by the ebb and flow of our feelings. They may range from ecstasy to despair, intense frustration to calm, to emptiness, loneliness, frustration, and anger within a single day. It is perhaps this variety of inner experience that provides the richness of our lives.

Many of us learn to fear our feelings in childhood—either by example, like seeing other people cry or be hurt, or through instruction, as in: "Big boys don't cry," "Don't express anger in this family," "If you're lonely, that's your problem."

Food, that universal panacea, is always available to help out. It seems always to comfort, never says no, and fills that inner emptiness.

Think about it for a minute. How often do you eat when you feel stressed, anxious, bored, sad, alone, depressed, happy, frustrated, excited, speeded up, or when you're suffering from insomnia or headaches, having difficulty concentrating, or when you're just plain upset? Food would be the ideal medicine were it not for the side effect of weight gain.

Everyone uses it every day for many purposes, few of which are related to nutritional needs. This is a universal human trait, not a habit of just the overweight.

Unfortunately, it is a source of unnecessary calories, and sets up the no-win situation where calories eaten to "deal with" an unpleasant feeling in turn lead to weight gain—which makes self-esteem worse, and creates an increasing sense of loss of control. Naturally, overeaters turn to food for more comfort. Eventually their self-esteem erodes, as more negative self-statements and putdowns creep into their thoughts about themselves. More problems are created by this type of eating than any medicine could ever treat.

For the overweight person who habitually eats in response to feelings, there is additional conditioning. A feeling state such as anxiety becomes associated with the desire to eat. This is the same type of conditioning as that of the person who habitually watches television and finds that her favorite television show makes her hungry: A simple learned response. The emotional eater finds that the emotion itself creates hunger.

The first step in breaking these patterns is awareness. It's okay to have feelings; in fact it would be abnormal to go through life with no feelings. The more you're aware of them, the easier they are to cope with. By feelings, we mean the entire range of human experience, from small shifts in mood during the day to the devastation of separation and divorce, loss of a loved one, failure on an examination or even a move to a new city.

Feelings *are* the human condition. However, feelings are *not* inevitably linked to eating.

HOMEWORK

This week the food dairy asks you to keep track of feelings that lead to eating, or feelings that in the past would have led to eating. If other intense emotional states come along that are unassociated with eating, write them down also. For example, if Monday you find yourself snacking on a piece of cheese at home because you're tired, frustrated, or angry after a hard day at work, jot that down. If on Tuesday, you're wishing that you had a candy bar, because that would make you feel better when you feel lonely, jot that down. If by Friday you're craving a bit of extra food because you "deserve it," and you've worked hard all week and haven't received any recognition, jot that down.

What we're interested in this week is feelings that in the past might have led to excess eating, currently do lead to excess eating, and feelings that you might in future "medicate" with a chocolate mousse.

The homework assignment for this week is:

A. This week you will concentrate on your emotional associations with eating. Keep track of each eating episode, and pay particular attention to accompanying feelings. Record them in this week's diary, and rate them as indicated on the food diary form.

B. Keep up the good work with your exercise and extra activity, and record them on the Daily Activity Record.

FOOD DIARY — Lesson Thirteen **Sample**

EATING URGES AND FEELINGS

On this diary, keep track of urges to eat on a scale of 0-10, with 0 being no urge, and 10 an almost irresistable urge to eat. At home, you might do this with actual eating episodes or snacks instead of urges to eat.

Day of Week ____________________ Date ____________________

Time	Urge (0-10)	Type of Food	Feeling State
6:00 7:15	2	Cereal, o.j	calm
10:15	0	sweet roll	frustrated
11:00 12:30	0	hamburger, ice cream	angry
4:00 4:15	0	Coffee, donut	tired
7:30	1	Pork chops	drained
9:00			tired

FOOD DIARY — Lesson Thirteen

EATING URGES AND FEELINGS

On this diary, keep track of urges to eat on a scale of 0-10, with 0 being no urge, and 10 an almost irresistable urge to eat. At home, you might do this with actual eating episodes or snacks instead of urges to eat.

Day of Week ______________ Date ______________

Time	Urge (0-10)	Type of Food	Feeling State
6:00			
11:00			
4:00			
9:00			

FOOD DIARY — Lesson Thirteen

EATING URGES AND FEELINGS

On this diary, keep track of urges to eat on a scale of 0-10, with 0 being no urge, and 10 an almost irresistable urge to eat. At home, you might do this with actual eating episodes or snacks instead of urges to eat.

Day of Week ____________________ Date ____________________

Time	Urge (0-10)	Type of Food	Feeling State
6:00			
11:00			
4:00			
9:00			

FOOD DIARY — Lesson Thirteen

EATING URGES AND FEELINGS

On this diary, keep track of urges to eat on a scale of 0-10, with 0 being no urge, and 10 an almost irrestistable urge to eat. At home, you might do this with actual eating episodes or snacks instead of urges to eat.

Day of Week ____________________ Date ____________________

Time	Urge (0-10)	Type of Food	Feeling State
6:00			
11:00			
4:00			
9:00			

FOOD DIARY — Lesson Thirteen

EATING URGES AND FEELINGS

On this diary, keep track of urges to eat on a scale of 0-10, with 0 being no urge, and 10 an almost irresistable urge to eat. At home, you might do this with actual eating episodes or snacks instead of urges to eat.

Day of Week ______________ Date ______________

Time	Urge (0-10)	Type of Food	Feeling State
6:00			
11:00			
4:00			
9:00			

FOOD DIARY — Lesson Thirteen

EATING URGES AND FEELINGS

On this diary, keep track of urges to eat on a scale of 0-10, with 0 being no urge, and 10 an almost irresistable urge to eat. At home, you might do this with actual eating episodes or snacks instead of urges to eat.

Day of Week ________________ Date ________________

Time	Urge (0-10)	Type of Food	Feeling State
6:00			
11:00			
4:00			
9:00			

FOOD DIARY — Lesson Thirteen

EATING URGES AND FEELINGS

On this diary, keep track of urges to eat on a scale of 0-10, with 0 being no urge, and 10 an almost irresistable urge to eat. At home, you might do this with actual eating episodes or snacks instead of urges to eat.

Day of Week ____________________ Date ____________________

Time	Urge (0-10)	Type of Food	Feeling State
6:00			
11:00			
4:00			
9:00			

FOOD DIARY — Lesson Thirteen

EATING URGES AND FEELINGS

On this diary, keep track of urges to eat on a scale of 0-10, with 0 being no urge, and 10 an almost irresistable urge to eat. At home, you might do this with actual eating episodes or snacks instead of urges to eat.

Day of Week ______________________ Date ______________________

Time	Urge (0-10)	Type of Food	Feeling State
6:00			
11:00			
4:00			
9:00			

DAILY ACTIVITY RECORD

(Fill in miles per day walked and minutes of exercise or extra activities)

	Monday		**Tuesday**		**Wednesday**		**Thursday**		**Friday**		**Saturday**		**Sunday**	
	Miles	**Calories**	**Miles**	**Calories**	**Miles**	**Calories**	**Miles**	**Calories**	**Miles**	**Calories**	**Miles**	**Calories**	**Miles**	**Calories**
Miles Walked														
Activity or Exercise	**Mins.**	**Calories**	**Mins.**	**Calories**	**Mins.**	**Calories**	**Mins.**	**Calories**	**Mins.**	**Calories**	**Mins.**	**Calories**	**Mins.**	**Calories**

Use the table on page 109 and 110 to calculate the caloric equivalent of each activity. If your activity is not included, chose one from the list that is similar.

LESSON FOURTEEN DEALING WITH FEELINGS— THINK BEFORE YOU BITE

WEIGH-IN AND HOMEWORK

For the fourteenth time, weigh yourself, record your weight on your Personal Weight Record, and graph your weight change. Record it here also:

weight on day 1______ weight today______

Pat yourself on the back for your work over 14 weeks to change your eating habits and increase your activity patterns. Pat yourself on the back for your weight loss.

REVIEW

Last week I introduced the concept of self-image. If, in your mind's eye, you remain overweight or fat or gross or "whale like," you won't have much of a chance of maintaining any weight loss. On the other hand, if you can visualize the future, suspend your judgment for a while, and allow what you want to be to become reality, your chances at maintenance will be much better.

You filled out a "Future Autobiography" last week. Turn back to it and read it over. This image, which you painted in words, will become a reality in time. It's an image that you need to keep in your mind's eye. Without this specific goal, you will have a difficult time keeping motivated over the months and years of maintenance.

When you did your Future Autobiography, did you have trouble with any of the topics? If so, this gives you clues about where you will run into problems in the future. For example, if you answered "my social life—dating—will be 'minimal because I don't have many friends,'" you have admitted to yourself that this is an area of your life that needs improvement. If your social life doesn't change, or if there probably won't be any dating after you lose weight and change your behaviors, pretty soon you will ask yourself, "why be thin?" You'll very rapidly turn to food for solace, and regain your weight.

Look at each of your answers critically. If necessary, redo your Future Autobiography every few weeks until a more hopeful image of yourself begins to crystalize.

In the second part of last week's lesson, you learned about the intimate relationship between food and feelings. Food is the universal medicine. It will sooth the most troubled person, brighten her up, slow her down, help her to sleep, give her energy to stay awake, calm her despair, and fill that empty, longing feeling inside. It's potent stuff. Unfortunately, the main side effect of this miraculous medicine is **fat.**

In your homework assignment you made a list of eating episodes associated with feelings, urges to eat associated with feelings, and any extra eating associated with feelings. Remember—an urge to eat that isn't counteracted by an alternate behavior becomes a snack—or a meal.

DEALING WITH FEELINGS

This next week, I want you to practice dealing with feelings in non-food-related ways. This week's food diary has a place to list any emotional episodes that could trigger eating, and the solutions that you develop for each particular feeling state.

This may happen once or twice a day, or once or twice a week. Keep track of as many of them as you can, and the solutions. Be creative. Although the list of feelings that can trigger eating in this lesson list only 10, remember there are many many more, and certainly more solutions than I have suggested.

Feelings That Can Trigger Eating

Feeling No. 1: Stressed out

Practice relaxation (you can read about relaxation in Lesson 15), go jogging, meditate, think about a pleasant time in the past, listen to music.

Feeling No. 2: Feeling anxious

Try relaxation exercises (see Lesson 15) or some physical activity. Make sure you aren't drinking excess coffee, tea, or other caffeinated beverages. Also make sure you aren't taking medication that makes you feel this way.

Feeling No. 3: Boredom

This is universal. It is best fought with a list of friends, list of alternate activities, a good book at hand, or something physical you can do.

Feeling No. 4: Loneliness

Give it a try with phone calls to friends and family, letter writing, a church group, Toastmasters, self-help organizations, and volunteer services.

Feeling No. 5: Depressed

Try to identify the source of the "downer"—a loss, separation, difference of opinion, perceived criticism, or unexpressed anger. Define it by describing it on paper, or talk it over with someone else. If it is a major loss, for example a divorce or a death, you might seek counseling.

Feeling No. 6: Frustration

Identify one source of your frustration and confront it—at work, with your spouse, with children, or in your neighborhood. State your wishes and desires clearly to resolve frustrating situations. Then move on to other sources of frustration.

Feeling No. 7: Feeling tired

Take a 10-minute nap, or go for a walk.

Feeling No. 8: Can't sleep

Try a warm bath, relaxation, or (if it works for you) even some tryptophan from the health food store.

Feeling No. 9: Hyperactivity

Try relaxation exercises. Are you driving yourself too hard, or is someone else pushing you into hyperactivity? Are you trying to avoid something?

Feeling No. 10: Aches and pains

How about some physical exercises, massage and heat, even a hot shower?

If there are some I have missed, list them below with possible solutions. Remember, we are all unique in our feelings—and free to add to all of these examples and work out solutions that fit our own life-styles. Remember also, the solutions should be food-free, and easily implemented so they can compete with food.

Take some time and care in looking at your feelings—you will need some of them analyzed to do this week's homework. This is one of those lessons that can be repeated, over and over—so if you need time to think about your feelings and their relationships to eating urges and snacks, or extra eating, take it.

Feeling No. 11: ______________________________

____

____

____

Feeling No. 12: ______________________________

____

____

____

Feeling No. 13: ______________________________

____

____

____

Feeling No. 14: ______________________________

____

____

____

Feeling No. 15: ______________________________

____

____

____

Make a list of the feelings that you identified on your food diary during the past week that caused strong urges to eat or actually led to "extra" eating. ______

______

______

______

______

______

______

______

______

Even though food temporarily takes care of most feelings, there are other ways of dealing with them. A list of alternate behaviors can provide a ready source of solutions. Read over your list of feelings and solutions, and compare it with the ones listed in this lesson. How do you compare? Did you develop some individual solutions that I did not list? What were they?

Behavioral Prescriptions: ______

______

______

______

NEW TOPIC: COGNITIVE RESTRUCTURING

We all talk to ourselves all the time. This doesn't mean we are crazy. We have repetitive thoughts, and an on-going internal dialogue about our surroundings and feelings throughout much of the day.

They can be positive and supportive. Or they can be negative and distressing. We are concerned here about both—you need all of the self support you can muster—and you need to change self-defeating internal dialogues.

To change self-defeating internal dialogues, it is necessary to modify your thought patterns. For example, if you always say to yourself, "I can't do it, I'm a fat slob, and no amount of dieting in the world will be successful," you won't do well with eating habit changes. Why should a fat slob change? She can't, almost by definition. Or, if you achieve a goal, for example eating in your designated eating place successfully, but never congratulate yourself, it won't be worth the effort. The new behavior will vanish very rapidly.

You can work with some of your negative feelings and attitudes, and change them into positives. For example, the feeling of being hungry is generally thought of as unpleasant. But if you can always think of it as the feeling of fat being burned off your body, it becomes more acceptable to be hungry some of the time. The feeling can be thought of as similar to the muscle tiredness you feel after you exercise. It's there for a reason. It's a mark of success. What coach hasn't told his team, "no pain, no gain!"

It is necessary to carefully assess repetitive thought patterns for negative self-commentary. If you find yourself constantly commenting on the negative, STOP—and ask yourself, "why am I being so negative?" For example, if you ate a little too much, instead of coming down hard on yourself, why not compliment yourself on your other successes and progress, instead of dwelling on the fact that you blew it a little bit on one occasion. The negative won't help—the little bit of positive feels good even when you've "blown it."

If you're the kind of person who sees the world as black and white, all or nothing, good or bad, success or failure, you are set-up for going on and off of diets the rest of your life. If you have to be perfect, you won't make it. Allow yourself to be human, allow yourself to cheat on the diet a little bit.

Let's stop for a minute and look at some sample "internal dialogues" and how to change them. These are typical rationalizations that we all use to "allow" or "justify" extra eating.

Rationalizations	Alternative Script
I have to eat. Everyone else is, and if I don't, they will be upset with me.	Sure, I have to eat, but I don't have to eat right now. I'm not hungry. I will eat when *I am* hungry, not when it is expected. I can still be with them and have a salad instead of a meal.

Rationalizations	Alternative Script
I blew it! It's all over! I blew it. I might as well really blow it. Where's the Hagen Daz?	So what! Everyone loses control once in a while. I'll start again right now. There is no point trying to "make up for it" with a lot of painful exercise or ice cream—that would probably make me feel sorry for myself and want to eat more. The best thing is to start over now.
My aunt says I shouldn't lose weight. My psychiatrist says I have enough going on now without worrying about eating. My husband says I'm not fun.	I need to make up my own mind and make my own choices. I'm not going to use other people's opinions as excuses for my own behavior. If they want to be fat, that's their decision.

These typical rationalizations have been paired with alternative statements on the right. In each case, the rationalization that would have led to extra eating has been replaced with a statement that kept the person in control of her eating, her weight, and her self-esteem.

What are some of your "excess eating scripts?" Write down a few on the left-hand side of the worksheet below, and re-write them on the right-hand side of the page.

My Rationalizations	My Alternative Script
1.	
2.	
3.	

If you practice replacing your rationalizations with alternative scripts, eventually the changes will come to you automatically.

Self-reinforcement, that pat on the back from yourself, is vital. For many, particularly those who live alone, this may be the only source of pats on the back. So when you've accomplished any of the behavioral, physical, or dietary tasks in this program, sit back and gloat a little. Tell yourself you did a *great* job.

HOMEWORK

A. Keep track of the miles per day you walk.

B. Once a day (or more) use the Script Writing form to change an excess eating rationalization to one that discourages extra eating—write it down.

C. Pat yourself on the back when you do things well—even little things. When you go to bed at night, reflect on the positives you have accomplished and admit to yourself that you've done a good, but admittedly not-perfect, job—that you are a pretty clever person.

D. Use the Urges, Snacks, Feelings, and Behaviors form to keep track of feelings that would formerly have led to eating. Write down how strong your urge was, once a day if possible, and think up a behavioral alternative. If it leads to a snack, write it down anyway, along with your feelings. Sometimes mistakes are our best teachers.

Lesson Fourteen

MILEAGE RECORD

	M	T	W	Th	F	S	S
Miles Walked Per Day							

Lesson Fourteen

Sample

SCRIPT WRITING

	Rationalization	Alternative Script
Mon	I have no will power, so I can't expect to control eating.	Everyone slips at times. I need more practise.
Tue	No one cares how I look.	I care how I look.
Wed	1 donut is only 100 calories	It is the "not very many calories" that add up.
Thurs	I need sweet snacks to "pick me up"	I do better with a relaxing break.
Fri	I can't help eating when I'm bored	I'll find a good book.
Sat	I've blown it, so I might as well hog up	Now's a time when it's really important to do something besides eating
Sun	I'd rather not go out on dates.	I'll work to feel good about my looks, and see how I feel about dates.

Lesson Fourteen

SCRIPT WRITING

	Rationalization	Alternative Script
Mon		
Tue		
Wed		
Thurs		
Fri		
Sat		
Sun		

Lesson Fourteen

SCRIPT WRITING

	Rationalization	Alternative Script
Mon		
Tue		
Wed		
Thurs		
Fri		
Sat		
Sun		

URGES, SNACKS, FEELINGS AND BEHAVIORS — Lesson Fourteen

Rate urges on a scale of 0-10. List alternative behaviors used even if they don't work.

Sample

Day of Week ____________________ Date ____________________

Time	Urge (0-10)	Snack	Feeling	Alternative Behavior Used
6:00				
11:00 11:30	10	cheesecake	anger	Tried Coffee break
4:00 8:00	6	—	Bored	Called a friend
9:00				

URGES, SNACKS, FEELINGS AND BEHAVIORS — Lesson Fourteen

Rate urges on a scale of 0-10. List alternative behaviors used even if they don't work.

Day of Week ______________________ Date ______________________

Time	Urge (0-10)	Snack	Feeling	Alternative Behavior Used
6:00				
11:00				
4:00				
9:00				

URGES, SNACKS, FEELINGS AND BEHAVIORS — Lesson Fourteen

Rate urges on a scale of 0-10. List alternative behaviors used even if they don't work.

Day of Week ____________ Date ____________

Time	Urge (0-10)	Snack	Feeling	Alternative Behavior Used
6:00				
11:00				
4:00				
9:00				

URGES, SNACKS, FEELINGS AND BEHAVIORS — Lesson Fourteen

Rate urges on a scale of 0-10. List alternative behaviors used even if they don't work.

Day of Week ____________________ Date ____________________

Time	Urge (0-10)	Snack	Feeling	Alternative Behavior Used
6:00				
11:00				
4:00				
9:00				

URGES, SNACKS, FEELINGS AND BEHAVIORS — Lesson Fourteen

Rate urges on a scale of 0-10. List alternative behaviors used even if they don't work.

Day of Week ____________________ Date ____________________

Time	Urge (0-10)	Snack	Feeling	Alternative Behavior Used
6:00				
11:00				
4:00				
9:00				

URGES, SNACKS, FEELINGS AND BEHAVIORS — Lesson Fourteen

Rate urges on a scale of 0-10. List alternative behaviors used even if they don't work.

Day of Week ______________ Date ______________

Time	Urge (0-10)	Snack	Feeling	Alternative Behavior Used
6:00				
11:00				
4:00				
9:00				

URGES, SNACKS, FEELINGS AND BEHAVIORS — Lesson Fourteen

Rate urges on a scale of 0-10. List alternative behaviors used even if they don't work.

Day of Week ____________________ Date ____________________

Time	Urge (0-10)	Snack	Feeling	Alternative Behavior Used
6:00				
11:00				
4:00				
9:00				

URGES, SNACKS, FEELINGS AND BEHAVIORS — Lesson Fourteen

Rate urges on a scale of 0-10. List alternative behaviors used even if they don't work.

Day of Week ____________________ Date ____________________

Time	Urge (0-10)	Snack	Feeling	Alternative Behavior Used
6:00				
11:00				
4:00				
9:00				

LESSON FIFTEEN

STRESS—THE SOFT UNDERBELLY OF FAT

WEIGH-IN AND HOMEWORK

Weigh yourself, calculate your weight loss for the past week, record and graph it on your Personal Weight Record.

- Last week I walked an average of______ miles per day.
- My baseline miles per day (Lesson Five, page 88) was______.
- I am walking______ miles more per day than I was back then.
- I intend to continue with my activity at this level or greater. Yes______ No______

REVIEW

Two weeks ago we reviewed self-image, and its vital importance to the long-term success of your weight control program. Your Future Autobiography helped you look at your self-image and at parts of that image that you would like to change.

- Do you remember reading this part of the book? Yes______ No______

- Are there still self-image issues that you need to clarify?
  Yes_______ No_______
  If so, try re-working Lessons Thirteen and Fourteen.

We then looked at an all too common pattern, eating when you are having strong feelings. These range from fatigue to anxiety to anger. Most of us, at some time in our life, learn that feelings are not as acceptable as eating, and we turn to the refrigerator for that marvelous medication called food. It can control any feeling, at least for a while.

You kept track of your feelings, and looked at some behavioral prescriptions for a variety of feeling states.

The Food Diaries for Lessons Thirteen and Fourteen included a place to jot down feelings, eating urges, and solutions.

- How many times when you had a strong feeling were you able to use one of the behavioral prescriptions you had thought up ahead of time to deal with your food-directed feeling?_______

- Did this save you any extra eating episodes?
  Yes_______ No_______

These behavioral prescriptions need not be limited to feelings that lead to excess weight. They are general techniques that are a part of everyday life. They are techniques that will help you cope with this increasingly complex world.

- Did you succeed fully and avoid any snacks by using your behavioral prescriptions last week?
  Yes_______ No_______

Last week we discussed thinking styles. We all talk to ourselves all the time. We have repetitive thought patterns, make repetitive comments about the world, and repeat repetitive excuses. If every time you approach food you say, "I'm a fat slob, I can't do it," no amount of dieting or behavioral management will be successful.

If, however, those negative *thoughts* about yourself and food can be turned around and become positive statements, the outcome will be far better. Even negative *feelings*, for example the feeling of hunger, can be changed or given a new meaning. It can be as simple as beginning to realize that the feeling of hunger, instead of being a terrible hardship, is the feeling of fat leaving your body. Hunger then is a more bearable feeling, because it is a sign of progress, much like muscle soreness is a sign of progress in a physical conditioning program.

Self-reinforcement is important in everyday life, just as it is in a dieting program. That pat on the back may not be forthcoming from someone else, so it's important to pat yourself on the back when you do something right. You might even use an outrageous compliment, like "you handsome, clever devil," or "you sexy man-killer."

Last week you kept track of your food-related rationaliz ations. It's impossible to write them all down, but even a few will give you a feeling for your "cognitive style." One of the examples I used was, "I have to eat because everyone else is eating, and if I don't, they will be upset with me." The alternative script suggested for that destructive rationalization was, "Sure I have to eat, but I don't have to eat right now. I'm not hungry. I'll eat when I am hungry, not when it is expected of me. I can resist that peer pressure. I can still be with them while they eat, and have a salad instead of a meal."

If you can develop a habit of catching yourself when you are making rationalizations, and start turning them around to less destructive or even supportive statements, you will soon automatically begin thinking in a thin style. Instead of trying to cover up extra eating with excuses, you'll prevent it by eliminating the self-defeating thought patterns that have allowed you to overeat and kept you from resisting food in the past.

- When you reviewed your homework today, were you surprised by any of your rationalizations?
  Yes______ No______

Many people feel self-conscious about changing even the most obvious rationalizations. Don't be shy—no one is looking. Now is the time to work on those excuses you have used for so many years.

NEW TOPIC: STRESS

All of us are exposed to stress every day. Stress has always been a part of the human condition. Without it to motivate us, we would have all been eaten by wolves, or even dinosaurs a long time ago.

Stress is not necessarily negative. For example, getting married is a stressful event, just as is divorce. Building a house is as stressful as selling a house. A promotion at work can be as stressful as losing your job. Stress indicates a departure from the status quo. Losing weight causes stress, as does changing body size, shape, and self image.

Stress is important in behavior change programs because of the tendency of people to eat when they feel themselves stressed. Food has an anxiety reducing, stress reducing, relaxing effect for many people. It doesn't matter whether the stress is positive or negative, or whether it's planned, like a new business venture, or unexpected, like a business loss. All types of stress can lead to excess eating.

Knowing this, you can look at your stressors. Can they be changed, or are they an essential part of your environment? If it's something you can't escape, such as the stress of work, or the stress of having a family, then you must learn to adapt to it, but without extra eating.

On the other hand, if a stressor is unnecessary—or irrelevant to your life and happiness, for example the stress of being on too many committees, then the obvious (although not always easy) solution is to get rid of some of your commitments.

There are many ways of dealing with stress besides eating. The oldest and perhaps the most effective is through relaxation. Although it may seem ironic, most people in our society do not know how to relax—they need to be taught how to do it!

We tend to think of relaxation as five minutes of sitting quietly, or watching a movie, or jogging. All of these can partially relax us. They nudge us in the direction of relaxation. They are calming, but they don't take us to the point where a physiologist would say, "this body is relaxed." Many times being calm isn't enough. You need to let all of your residual tension go.

Relaxation has many uses. In general, the more one is relaxed, the more appropriately one deals with stress (and inappropriate eating urges). The payoffs aren't restricted to food. They can be found throughout many areas of life—better business interactions, a calmer environment at home, and a reduction of blood pressure and lessening of stress related disease.

Stress reduction techniques, for example, deep muscle relaxation, can be used as an alternative to excess eating. When you have learned these techniques, you will be able, when you have the urge to eat, to simply take a few deep breaths, and let your body relax.

If you need to, you will be able to intensify the relaxation response simply be escaping into a world of fantasy, imagining for instance that you are in a relaxing place—like lying on a warm, sunny beach. When you need to, you will be able to take such one-or-two-minute "fantasy vacations" from the world around you, leaving the urges to eat behind. With practice, you will be able to use relaxation, and stress reduction techniques not only to deal with urges to eat, but also to deal with the overall stress quotient of your everyday life.

RELAXATION TECHNIQUES

Progressive Muscle Relaxation

There are several different ways to induce a state of profound relaxation. The grandfather technique of all is progressive muscle relaxation, invented by Dr. Jacobson at the University of Chicago in 1928. His technique teaches relaxation by letting go of induced tension. The technique is called progressive, because it proceeds through all of the major muscle groups in the body, tensing them and then relaxing them, one at a time.

This technique is time consuming, but it works. It has stood the test of time. Although the instructions initially can seem tedious, with practice they can be condensed to the point where a person can take a few deep breaths, breathe out while saying the word "relax," and let all of the tension flow out of his body. It also has the advantage that people who have specific areas of tension, for example, the neck, can relieve themselves of the tension by contracting the muscles that are involved, and then letting the tension flow out of the muscle group.

To be successful, relaxation must be practiced. When it is, the effects can be quite significant. Studies done at Stanford University have shown that this technique can lower the blood pressure of hypertensive patients to the point where some can stop using medication.

The following instructions are easiest to follow if they are read on to a tape recorder, and then played back.

Arrange for some quiet time, when you will not be interrupted by telephones, people, dogs, or extraneous sounds. Find a comfortable place to sit or lie down, and make yourself comfortable. Take a few deep breaths, and when you feel comfortable, close your eyes.

Now, to become aware of the differences between tension and relaxation, clench your right fist. Hold it tighter and tighter, and focus on the tension that develops in the muscles of your fist and forearm. Keep it tense until the muscles begin to quiver—and then let go, and observe the contrast in feeling between the tense, uptight feeling when you clenched your fist, and the feeling of relaxation and warmth when you let go. Now, try this again. Notice the difference once more. Next, repeat the process by clenching your left fist, clench it tightly until it begins to quiver, then relax. Notice the contrast between the tense feeling and the relaxed feeling. Now clench both fists tighter and tighter—then let the tension go.

Relax for a minute, and then tense your forearms and biceps on both sides. Hold the tension until all of these muscles begin to quiver, forearm, biceps and even the triceps on the back side of the arm. Then let go. Let the tension flow out, and feel the warmth as relaxation takes the place of tension. Pay close attention to those feelings.

Now, push your shoulders together in front of you, and feel the tension as you try to touch your shoulders together.

The tension is through your neck and back. Pull your shoulders up toward your head, toward your ears, and you will feel a different set of muscles become tense. Then drop your shoulders and let them relax. Let the tension flow out of your shoulders and neck region. Then try to touch your shoulders behind your back—try for about five seconds and then let go to relax again.

Now switch your attention to the other end of your body. Press your toes and feet downward away from your face, so that the calf muscles become tense and quiver. Then let go and feel the warmth as both calf muscles unwind. Push your toes downward, curl them under your feet, and at the same time pull your toes upward toward your knee cap. Hold that uncomfortable tense position as long as you can, and let go. You will find a warmth in your toes, the balls of your feet, and front of your legs.

Next try tensing the inside muscles of your legs by putting your feet together and pushing them together towards each other. Feel the muscles tense all along your legs, and possibly up into your eye muscles, then let go. Then flex your buttocks and thighs by tightening up, to the point where you begin to lift yourself out of your seat. It helps to press down on your heels as hard as you can. At this point, you are tensing the largest muscle groups in your body, and your whole body may begin to quiver. When you can no longer hold the tension, let go, sink back into the chair, and feel the process of relaxation overriding the residual feeling of tension.

Next push your knees together, and you will feel a different set of muscles tense. For completeness, you can try holding your knees together with your hands and pushing apart with your knees to tense the final set of muscles in the thighs. When you let go, your feet, toes, ankles, calves and thighs should be quite relaxed.

Now for a minute or two, just take some deep breaths, and enjoy the relaxation that you have induced. Then move your tension up to your abdominal area, and tighten your stomach muscles. Make your abdomen hard by pulling the muscles in, then push them out—and relax. Notice the contrast between the tension and the relaxation when you pull in. Do it again. Push out, and let go.

Now, move your attention to your lower back. Arch your back and make the tension appear along your spine. If necessary, move your shoulder blades back until they almost touch. Try to keep the rest of your body, particularly the part you've already worked on, from getting tense. Try to localize the tension throughout your lower back, and all the way up the spine—then let go. Try this several times, and then try tensing and relaxing your stomach once more. By now, most of the muscle groups of your body have been relaxed.

Now move your attention up to your head, and try tensing your forehead by gazing upwards and making wrinkles. Keep it as tense as you can, and then relax. Now frown, increase your brows, and study the tension in these muscles, and then relax. Try making a large grin, and clench your jaws at the same time. Study the tension. This spreads down into your neck and up towards your ears. As you do this, you can even hear the tension in your ears. Now let go of these tense muscles, and let the relaxation flow in.

Close your eyes very hard until you see stars. Try tightening your eye lids as tightly as possible, and then relax them and let the tension flow away. You can even relax the eye muscles themselves by first gazing up with your eyes shut, then to the left, then to the right, and then down. Then let your eyes return to their neutral, relaxed position. If you hold each position of the eye muscles for four or five seconds, you can become aware of the tension you generate by doing this, and the good feeling as the eye returns to center.

Next, try feeling relaxation all over your head. You can even relax your tongue, by pushing it first against the top of your mouth and then down against the bottom of your mouth, and then all the way to the right, and then all the way to the left. Then let it return to normal.

Many people can become aware of the wave of tension and relaxation that goes with swallowing. But for people who suffer occasional spasms of the esophagus, sometimes it is helpful to practice taking a drink of water and holding it in your mouth then slowly swallowing and following the course of the fluid down your esophagus, and into your stomach. If you use cold water, it will allow you to track the progress of the water more closely.

Finally, bring your attention back to your chest. Take a deep breath, hold it, and study the tension in your diaphragm and in the muscles between your ribs. Then let the tension go, and study that feeling. Do this four or five times, alternating a deep breath, and holding it, and then allowing the breathing to return to neutral. You can also study the opposite effect by breathing out more than you normally would, holding that position for a few seconds, and then letting yourself breathe normally.

Review the tension throughout your body. If there are any muscle groups that seem to still be tense, or tighter than you would like, tense them as much as you can for four or five seconds, and then let go and let the tension flow out of them. As you get more and more relaxed, become aware of your breathing. Try to make your breathing as regular and rhythmic as normal, but a little deeper, with a little bit longer breaths. Enjoy this relaxed state.

After a while, the progressive muscle relaxation instructions can be reduced to the point of relaxing only, or even just taking a few deep breaths, locating any sites of tension, tensing those muscles, and then letting the tension flow out of your body.

Imaging

The second relaxation technique is positive imagery or visualization. It is necessary to be in a semi-relaxed state to begin with. The purpose of visualization is to transport you in your mind's eye to a pleasant, relaxing situation, for example, lying on the beach, under the sun, feeling the nice warm sand beneath you. You are in an extremely relaxed state, with no worries, and no interruptions. You can feel the sun beating down. You are sort of sleepy. You can hear the surf in the distance, with an occasional sea gull flying overhead. You can even feel a slight breeze as you relax.

Each person can make up three or four scenes like this, that take between two and five minutes to "get into." The more real, the more vivid the escape, the better the relaxation response. It becomes a positive daydream, in which you shut out the world, shut out the stress, shut out the telephone, and shut out the food. It is a needed mini-vacation that serves as an alternative to eating.

Autogenic Training

A third type of relaxation is autogenic training, a state of self-hypnosis, or self-induced relaxation. It is based on the concept of passively telling yourself that you are becoming more and more relaxed. Instead of just saying "relax," however, a physical metaphor is used—that of feeling heavier and heavier, or lighter and lighter. For most people, a sense of heaviness goes with a feeling of being relaxed.

You first sit in a chair or lie down, as with progressive muscle relaxation. You take a few deep breaths, and try to shut out the stress of the world. Then repeat to yourself, slowly, three or four times: *my right arm is heavy . . . my left arm is heavy . . . both of my arms are heavy . . . my neck is heavy . . . my head is heavy . . . my shoulders, neck and head are all heavy. I can feel the weight of my body pushing into the chair. My left leg is heavy . . . my calf is heavy . . . my left leg, calf and foot are all pressing down into the chair and into the floor. My right leg is heavy . . . my right calf is heavy . . . my right foot is heavy . . . my right foot, calf and thigh are all heavy and pushing down into the floor. I feel a warmth in all of my body parts, a warmth on my arm, a warmth on my hands, a warmth on my back, a warmth pressing on to my shoulders, a warmth in my head, a warmth that goes down my spine into my thighs, into my legs, into my feet.*

At the end of several minutes of autogenic training, some type of "re-entry" process is usually suggested. Usually this is accomplished by breathing slowly and deeply, and on the inhalation, saying a phrase or word like "I am calm, I am serene, I am relaxed." After doing this ten or fifteen times, you should feel quite relaxed.

Breathing exercises

A final relaxation technique combines breathing exercises, and simply trying to focus one's mind away from the stress of life, and the stress contained in your body. The technique is quite simple, but needs a space and time where there won't be any interruption.

Get relaxed in your favorite chair, and begin by shutting your eyes, and taking a few deep breaths. Try breathing using all of your lungs and your diaphragm, and holding your breath for a few seconds, then exhaling slowly and completely. As you adopt an almost square pattern of breathing, with a long, deep inhalation, a period of holding your breath, and a long period of exhalation, then holding your breath out, try to focus your closed eyes on a spot, perhaps a foot to eighteen inches in front of your nose.

With this combination of deep breathing and focusing attention, you can become quite adept at relaxing in a relatively short period of time, unless there are specific areas of tension in your body that don't "give way" to this type of technique. An advantage of this technique is that you can do it any time, any place, very unobtrusively.

It doesn't matter which of these techniques you use, they all work quite well, and are quite effective.

HOMEWORK

This week's food diary again has very little to do with food. I want you to keep using the forms you filled in for the last session to keep track of: (A) Negative feelings that you were able to head off with some type of behavioral prescription; and (B) Unrealistic rationalizations about eating, with a note about how you corrected them. In addition, you are to record, on a day-by-day basis, a measure of your stress.

The stress scale goes from 0 to 10. 0 is totally calm, at ease in the world, with no sense of tension. 10 is stressful to the point of feeling your muscles tightening, your stomach knotting up, and possibly other physical symptoms like palpatations, sweatiness, a tight constricted band around your chest, a rapid heart rate, or a feeling that you want to scream.

Most of us experience stress somewhere along this spectrum every day. For this exercise, however, try to come up with an average for four segments of the day: morning before work; starting work up until lunch; from the beginning of the afternoon until after dinner; and evening. By breaking down your day in this way you will develop an awareness of your daily stress pattern. This will help you pinpoint your stress—and the best times to use stress reduction techniques.

Remember that stress is totally subjective. Don't worry if your rating for Monday is different from your rating for Friday. all I care is that you just develop a scale for self-monitoring your stress, and then learn to use appropriate relaxation techniques.

The final part of the homework is to practice relaxation. Set aside 15 minutes when it's calm, when there is no one around, when there will be no interruptions. Make yourself comfortable, and try to let all the tension flow out of your body, breathing deeply. Shut everything else out of your mind, and just concentrate on letting go and relaxing.

At the end of your relaxation period, jot down your overall level of stress during your relaxation period on the same 0-10 scale, and compare it with your average for the day. Relaxation does make a difference. It feels good to take a few minutes off, to let some of that tension go from your life. More to the point, it reduces your tendency toward snacking and extra eating.

The homework assignment for this week is:

A. Urges, Snacks, Feelings and Behaviors Form

B. Script Writing

C. Stress Monitoring Record

URGES, SNACKS, FEELINGS AND BEHAVIORS — Lesson Fifteen

Rate urges on a scale of 0-10. List alternative behaviors used even if they don't work.

Day of Week ____________________ Date ____________________

Time	Urge (0-10)	Snack	Feeling	Alternative Behavior Used
6:00				
11:00				
4:00				
9:00				

URGES, SNACKS, FEELINGS AND BEHAVIORS — Lesson Fifteen

Rate urges on a scale of 0-10. List alternative behaviors used even if they don't work.

Day of Week ____________________ Date ____________________

Time	Urge (0-10)	Snack	Feeling	Alternative Behavior Used
6:00				
11:00				
4:00				
9:00				

URGES, SNACKS, FEELINGS AND BEHAVIORS — Lesson Fifteen

Rate urges on a scale of 0-10. List alternative behaviors used even if they don't work.

Day of Week ______________ Date ______________

Time	Urge (0-10)	Snack	Feeling	Alternative Behavior Used
6:00				
11:00				
4:00				
9:00				

URGES, SNACKS, FEELINGS AND BEHAVIORS — Lesson Fifteen

Rate urges on a scale of 0-10. List alternative behaviors used even if they don't work.

Day of Week ____________________ Date ____________________

Time	Urge (0-10)	Snack	Feeling	Alternative Behavior Used
6:00				
11:00				
4:00				
9:00				

URGES, SNACKS, FEELINGS AND BEHAVIORS — Lesson Fifteen

Rate urges on a scale of 0-10. List alternative behaviors used even if they don't work.

Day of Week ____________________ Date ____________________

Time	Urge (0-10)	Snack	Feeling	Alternative Behavior Used
6:00				
11:00				
4:00				
9:00				

URGES, SNACKS, FEELINGS AND BEHAVIORS — Lesson Fifteen

Rate urges on a scale of 0-10. List alternative behaviors used even if they don't work.

Day of Week ____________________ Date ____________________

Time	Urge (0-10)	Snack	Feeling	Alternative Behavior Used
6:00				
11:00				
4:00				
9:00				

URGES, SNACKS, FEELINGS AND BEHAVIORS — Lesson Fifteen

Rate urges on a scale of 0-10. List alternative behaviors used even if they don't work.

Day of Week ______________________ Date ______________________

Time	Urge (0-10)	Snack	Feeling	Alternative Behavior Used
6:00				
11:00				
4:00				
9:00				

Lesson Fifteen

SCRIPT WRITING

	Rationalization	Alternative Script
Mon		
Tue		
Wed		
Thurs		
Fri		
Sat		
Sun		

Lesson Fifteen

Sample

STRESS MONITORING RECORD

0= Calm
10= Ready to Scream

	Early Morning	Morning thru Lunch	Afternoon thru Dinner	Evening	Before Relaxation Practice	After Relaxation Practice
Mon	0	1	5	5	5	1
Tue	0	1	6	7	7	1
Wed	0	5	8	7	7	0
Thurs	0	1	3	3	3	0
Fri	0	1	3	3	3	0
Sat	0	1	1	0	0	0
Sun	0	1	1	1	1	0

Lesson Fifteen

STRESS MONITORING RECORD

0= Calm
10= Ready to Scream

	Early Morning	Morning thru Lunch	Afternoon thru Dinner	Evening	Before Relaxation Practice	After Relaxation Practice
Mon						
Tue						
Wed						
Thurs						
Fri						
Sat						
Sun						

LESSON SIXTEEN

COUPLES—IS YOUR FAMILY FATTENING?

WEIGH-IN AND HOMEWORK

Weigh yourself, record and graph your weight. My total weight loss for the 16 weeks has been______.

REVIEW

The last four weeks we have reviewed a number of psychological concepts. We began with self-image, and some topics related to self-esteem. We examined internal dialogues and the irrational processes that allow us to eat when we're not hungry, as well as the rationalizations that allow us to have convenient lapses in self-control. Finally, last week we talked about stress and eating. For homework you reviewed the past lessons, and spent some time rating your stress levels throughout the week.

Stress goes hand in hand with modern life. Some is imposed by outside sources like bills and buses. Other sources are internal, like perfection and performance. We need stress to live—but too much interferes with our lives, both physically with stress-related disease, and psychologically with a constant feeling of anxiety or tension.

We can control it, but to do this we have to take the time to learn and practice stress reduction skills. Last week we learned:

1. Relaxation techniques
2. How to monitor our stress levels throughout the day
3. The importance of relaxation PRACTICE

This week we will continue the relaxation exercises as a part of the homework. Relaxation will be of limited help at first. The real benefit comes after weeks of practice—when you become automatically more relaxed, almost by reflex, when you encounter a stressful situation.

For example, you might be expecting a phone call that would ordinarily be quite stressful. Instead of feeling helplessly anxious, when you hear the phone ring, you are able to take a few deep breaths, tell yourself to relax with each exhalation, and to get through the experience far more calmly and easily. Or you might come into the kitchen tense, and catch yourself heading for the refrigerator, and stop and practice relaxation. Or you might know that when the kids come home at 3:00, you tend to be tense and snack-and learn to relax ahead of time to prepare for their arrival.

NEW TOPIC: THE SOCIAL ENVIRONMENT—SPOUSE, FAMILY, AND FRIENDS

Is Your Family Involved in Your Program?

- Have your family members tried the behavior change techniques you have been learning?
  Yes______ No______

- Do you think they appreciate the amount of work and effort that goes into modifying a behavior as basic as eating?
  Yes______ No______

- Has anyone in your family or among your friends lost weight as a result of your effort?
  Yes______ No______

Couples

Over the years most couples and families get into a rigid pattern of eating: They have a relatively limited choice of foods, eat at the same time and place, and rarely change what has become a comfortable way of interacting. When one person diets, this pattern is disrupted. This can be unpleasant for the partner or family and, in trying to get back to the old way of doing things, may lead to subtle attempts to undermine the attempt at dieting. Often a dieting/exercise program is seen as an imposition.

In contrast, research shows that couples and families who resist this tendency, and lose weight together, or in which the weight loss by one member is firmly supported by the another, maintain the weight loss much more effectively. In families where the entire family is involved in the weight loss program, the outcome is better still.

If you have a partner (and he didn't start this program with you), stop and clarify your mutual expectations with respect to this program. If there are significant reasons why your weight loss efforts will be difficult for your partner, the problem should be discussed, and an understanding reached now, rather than ignoring the problem or trying to "get around" it. The ideal is for both of you to be losing weight at the same time, or at least to be on the same diet and eating the same types of foods.

In any weight loss program, there are many parts that can be shared by another, and even by the whole family. These include a discussion of menus, and an emphasis on the importance of making calorically dense foods unavailable, e.g., the mid-afternoon snacks of the teenagers, as well as the late night snack of the husband.

There is nothing wrong with everyone in the family eating the same type of food (though not necessarily the same amounts). There's nothing more frustrating than being on a weight loss program, and finding that during the last shopping trip no low-calorie snacks were purchased, leaving you with only the kids' snacks in the middle of the night. Unless everyone supports your diet program, it is doomed to failure.

If each partner is able to help the other, to monitor each others' eating behaviors, activity, and exercise programs, a feeling of comradery and teamwork builds, and the weight loss progresses more smoothly. To the extent that this can be facilitated by talking with one another, family discussions, and family events planned around something other than eating, the more successful it is.

Remember that love and food are not the same thing, that there are other ways to celebrate than edible "treats"—for example, a show, a weekend with someone else doing the chores or watching the children, a peaceful walk together in the evening (instead of a television show with beer and pretzels).

Family Reactions That Make it Harder for You

Families, spouses, and groups of friends have different styles of reacting to someone losing weight. However, there seem to be some patterns of interaction that are common. Interactions that are painful to the person who is trying to lose can be avoided, if they are anticipated and strategies are worked out in advance for coping with them.

These interactions do not occur because people are bad, evil, or mean. They occur because the people involved are not fully conscious of them or the harmful effects they can have. They are habitual ways of interacting, and they persist because there has never been sufficient reason to learn a new way to interact with one another.

Some of the most common feelings, through the eyes of the person trying to lose weight, are:

1. "No one seems to be interested in what I'm doing or in changing their own habits; others have bad eating habits and do not seem to care."
2. "My attempts to change are not supported; they are even ridiculed. Often people say the wrong things. They do not mean to hurt my feelings, but they do."
3. "I am discouraged, belittled, made to feel different, and even the brunt of jokes. People tease me about my weight even though I am changing and losing; it makes me want to say 'what the hell' ..."
4. "My efforts to change are ignored; my family and friends are always pessimistic, often despite my success."
5. "My loss of weight is praised, but when I try to maintain my weight loss and behavior change, they seem to forget and withdraw their support."
6. "I feel like I am being sabotaged; it is obvious to me, but I can't do anything about it:
   a. They give me high-calorie treats and presents;
   b. They insist I have high-calorie treats for them or the children;
   c. They continue the same old pattern—togetherness is an evening out with a good meal—we cannot be together without food;
   d. They bring me food at inappropriate times, like while I am watching TV;
   e. They use food as a sign of affection; it puts me in a bind;
   f. They say I'm becoming too skinny or unhealthy."

The reasons for these reactions are numerous. We can only guess about them. Some family members may not want to have to match your self-control, especially if they weigh too much themselves. They may not want things to change. They may be afraid that when you look nicer you will go away or run away with someone else, or they won't have anything to complain about.

However, the most probable explanation is that this is the only way they have learned to interact with you. It is the way that has worked in the past. It is a type of behavior neither one of you has been fully aware of. Fortunately, it is a behavior that is quite amenable to change.

To break out of these stereotyped interactions, the person losing weight—*you*—must take control of the situation. The people around you cannot really read your mind; they have to be told what you want. After all you are altering the relationship by losing weight, looking different, and feeling different about yourself. They need to know how to give you feedback and praise. So—

- Ask for support.
- Ask for praise. A compliment at the right time will go further than any material reward, be it money or cream puffs.
- Ask for feedback and thank them for it.

Remember, many of the behaviors you are changing are hard to detect. Many of your new habits are "non-behaviors," like *not* eating rapidly, or *not* eating in many different places. People around you will not intuitively know to compliment you for *eating less* or *not* finishing everything on your plate, unless they know your goals.

If this program is to succeed, and if you expect to lose weight and maintain that weight loss, then those behaviors must have positive consequences. They have to pay off! You must feel like it has been worth it. If your family and friends have been directly involved in the process of your weight loss, your success is also their success. Your mutual life will be better, and probably longer.

What You Can Do

The following suggestions are designed to help you involve others in the Maintenance part of your behavior change program, to make sure that weight loss and Maintenance pay off for you:

1. Ask for what you want—praise, feedback, cooperation, and rewards.
2. Request help with the techniques—those close to you can remind you of them or even experiment with them. Be in it together. If you practice together, you will do better.

3. Request that affection and sharing *not* be in terms of food. You may appreciate a huge gooey chocolate cake for your birthday, but other gifts are more appropriate. When you are offered a "food gift," you are put in a difficult situation. How can you turn down the gift without feeling like you are turning down the affection also? Try to establish the habit of using non-food treats, like flowers or activities, for celebrations.

4. Request that no one in your environment offer you food at any time. They should assume that if you want food, you will ask for it. Being offered food is a very strong social cue for eating—we all feel bad saying "no."

5. Try to minimize food topics in your conversation with friends and family during your period of weight loss. Discuss the program and progress, but request that they not talk about food. Talk about the office picnic or a good recipe are cues for eating.

6. Try to entertain without high-calorie foods. This takes cooperation from everyone. Friends will still visit you despite the lack of potato chips. If they want food, have low-calorie snacks available.

7. If your husband, children, or other significant person eats or snacks a great deal of the time, ask them to try not to do it around you. Watching someone else eat is a very strong cue to eat.

8. Try to develop exercise programs with another person. Companionship makes exercise more fun, makes it a social commitment to exercise, and gives you a non-food social activity.

Do You See the Importance of These Points?

- Do you see the importance of support by family and friends for your behavior change program? Yes______ No______

- Do you understand that no one is to blame for these patterns of interaction, that these are just habits which have developed over the years? Yes______ No______

- Did any of the common interpersonal reactions sound familiar? Yes______ No______

- Do you run into additional patterns repeatedly?
  Yes______ No______

- Are there any additional rules that should be added to the list for your social environment? Yes______ No______

  ____

  ____

  ____

HOMEWORK

If you are involved in a relationship, or family, I want you to include them in your weight loss program this week. Sit down with them, and have them choose one of the techniques from the previous 15 weeks to help you with, and to practice themselves. On the Cooperation Checklist, you'll find a place for them to check off every day, the statement "I was involved."

See if you can generate some comradery in your weight loss program. Up until now it's been a one-person show. The more you can involve those around you, the better your chances for keeping weight loss permanent.

In addition, I want you to continue working with the stress reduction techniques outlined in Lesson Fifteen, and to keep a Stress Monitoring Record.

Finally, at the end of the lesson you will find copies of an old friend—the original food diary form. I want you to fill it in for just Friday, Saturday and Sunday of this week.

The homework assignment for this week is:

A. Stress Monitoring Record

B. Cooperation Checklist

C. Food Diary

Lesson Sixteen

STRESS MONITORING RECORD

0= Calm
10= Ready to Scream

	Early Morning	Morning thru Lunch	Afternoon thru Dinner	Evening	Before Relaxation Practice	After Relaxation Practice
Mon						
Tue						
Wed						
Thurs						
Fri						
Sat						
Sun						

Lesson Sixteen

Sample

COOPERATION CHECKLIST

	Technique(s) Tried Together	Persons Involved (family/friend/spouse)
		husband
Mon	Eating in appropriate place	I was involved
Tue	Only eating	I was involved
Wed	Planned eating	I was involved
Thur	Fork: bite ratio	I was involved
Fri	Food out of sight	I was involved
Sat	Relaxation techniques	I was involved
Sun	Planned Shopping	I was involved

Lesson Sixteen

COOPERATION CHECKLIST

	Technique(s) Tried Together	Persons Involved (family/friend/spouse)
Mon		
Tue		
Wed		
Thur		
Fri		
Sat		
Sun		

FOOD DIARY — Lesson Sixteen

Friday, Saturday and Sunday only

Day of Week ____________________ Date ____________________

Time	Minutes Spent Eating	M/S	H	Body Position	Activity While Eating	Location of Eating	Kind of Food
6:00							
11:00							
4:00							
9:00							

M/S: Meal or Snack; H: Degree of Hunger (0 = None, 1 = Some, 2 = Normal, 3 = Good Healthy Hunger, 4 = Ravenous); Body Position: 1 = Walking, 2 = Standing, 3 = Sitting, 4 = Lying Down

FOOD DIARY — Lesson Sixteen

Friday, Saturday and Sunday only

Day of Week ________________ Date ________________

Time	Minutes Spent Eating	M/S	H	Body Position	Activity While Eating	Location of Eating	Kind of Food
6:00							
11:00							
4:00							
9:00							

M/S: Meal or Snack; H: Degree of Hunger (0 = None, 1 = Some, 2 = Normal, 3 = Good Healthy Hunger, 4 = Ravenous); Body Position: 1 = Walking, 2 = Standing, 3 = Sitting, 4 = Lying Down

FOOD DIARY — Lesson Sixteen

Friday, Saturday and Sunday only

Day of Week ____________________ Date ____________________

Time	Minutes Spent Eating	M/S	H	Body Position	Activity While Eating	Location of Eating	Kind of Food
6:00							
11:00							
4:00							
9:00							

M/S: Meal or Snack; H: Degree of Hunger (0 = None, 1 = Some, 2 = Normal, 3 = Good Healthy Hunger, 4 = Ravenous); Body Position: 1 = Walking, 2 = Standing, 3 = Sitting, 4 = Lying Down

LESSON SEVENTEEN

BEHAVIORAL ANALYSIS AND PROBLEM SOLVING— THE KEY TO SELF-HELP

WEIGH-IN AND HOMEWORK

Weigh yourself and record your weight and graph it on your Personal Weight Record. By now you should be patting yourself on the back quite frequently. Your weight loss is something to be proud of.

REVIEW

Last week we introduced your loved ones to your weight loss program. They were (circle one)

1. Enthusiastic
2. Negative
3. Lukewarm
4. Could care less
5. Other______________________________

The people around you are powerful forces in your behavioral change program. They can make it much easier—or much more difficult. If you feel their support, and love, you will have a much easier time of it than if you feel like you're out on a limb by yourself. With some couples, it is worse than that. It is not uncommon for some people to feel that if they change too much, their spouse/partner will abandon them.

Weight loss has to be for yourself. No one else can do it for you. However, the support of others certainly helps, and their lack of support or sabotage hurts. Talk with them about it—and about your fears.

As you have discovered, there is nothing wrong with everyone in the family eating the same type of food, even if it means Johnny has to give up his high-calorie yummies, and Susie her chocolate truffles.

In Lesson Nine when I talked about preplanning and shopping, you probably experienced some frustration when you discovered that whoever did the shopping forgot to buy the low-calorie foods. This left you stuck with the kids' sugary cereal in the middle of the night, instead of an apple or a banana. This sort of experience illustrates why communication is important in this program. Ask for help—let them know what you are doing. After sixteen weeks in the program, if someone is still offering you chocolate mousse cake for dessert every night, you haven't been communicating very well!

NEW TECHNIQUE: PROBLEM SOLVING, OR BECOMING YOUR OWN THERAPIST

The problems we have worked on up to now are universal; everyone with a weight problem has them. The solutions we have suggested are general and useful for everyone.

This week I want you to learn how to identify and solve your particular problems: to become your own weight management therapist. When you have finished, and the support of this program is no longer available, you will need the ability to spot your own eating problems and to solve them. Everyone has some problem eating behaviors which are unique, and some new ones will develop in the future—it is inevitable. However, if you apply the techniques taught here, you will have the skills to solve any eating problem.

We are all confronted with problems through most of our waking hours. Some of these are solved automatically—or with little thought. What should I wear? What am I going to do today? What time is dinner? Other problems, in particular those associated with diet, need to be carefully defined if you are to be successful at managing them.

The steps in solving behavioral problems are separated into five categories:

1. *Observation and Long-term Goal Definition.* This means

looking at the big problem to try to see what can be arranged. An example is using a food diary to look at eating behaviors, with an over-all goal of losing weight.

2. *Identification and Definition of Specific Well-Defined Objectives, or Short-term Goal Setting.* These objectives are the small steps you take toward a long-term goal. Each step is to be taken in connection with the behaviors you have identified during your observations; for example, looking at your food diary and identifying the habit of eating too large a breakfast, and considering the concrete steps you might take to change the habit.

3. *Creative Problem Solving, or Brainstorming.* This is a method of uncritically suggesting solutions to the defined problem. There are usually many ways to solve behavioral problems. No way is necessarily right or wrong; some ways are more direct, some faster, but many can be effective. For example, several techniques might be used to modify the habit of a large daily breakfast. I might propose:

   a. Slow down, and introduce a two-minute delay after the toast and coffee;

   b. Eliminate cues—for example, by eating only at the breakfast table (not at the open refrigerator), and not reading the paper at breakfast;

   c. Substitute lower-calorie foods—for example, artificial sweetners, thinner bread, and non-fat milk;

   d. Elimination techniques—for example, eliminating a food like bacon, or slowly decreasing the portion size of a food like bread. An almost endless list can be made for any specific problem. Most of the time several techniques can be used at the same time.

4. *Decision Making.* At this point, you choose and implement the plan or plans that seem to be most appropriate. In general, try to change behaviors only a few steps at a time. It is important not to go too fast or to change too many things at one time; you'll fail and become discouraged when things don't change. You should plan to succeed at least 80 percent of the time.

5. *Feedback and Evaluation.* This is one of the most important steps. If you do not periodically evaluate your progress, you will not know what works and what doesn't. If you find your plan is not working, don't charge yourself with lack of will

power or a moral defect; more likely, you didn't choose a good plan, or it is too big a change for one step, or perhaps you have not properly identified the problem. Look over the whole problem-solving process again, and don't be afraid to change plans if something isn't working. Be creative in your approach.

Reward. Deciding on a reward is not really part of the problem-solving process (so it isn't counted as a sixth step), but it's vitally important for the over-all success of your efforts. So make sure you think ahead, while you are still in the planning stage about a reward that you really will enjoy.

Observation

The first step is to get an idea of the general problem area, and the related behaviors. You need to reduce the problem to its essentials. This narrowing down of the problem comes from analyzing data. For example: I eat in too many places; I eat pizza four times a week; I seem to have 12 eating episodes a day (including each small snack or nibble when I go through the kitchen); or I'm not able to stick to my exercise program on the weekends. All of these problems are more specific than "I'm too fat" or "I eat too much."

In order to effectively narrow down a problem to its specific elements, an awareness of the events that precede and follow the particular event is important. For example, for snacking multiple times a day, the preceding event could be walking through the kitchen and seeing food, or feeling stressed and going to the kitchen and eating, or preparing snacks for the children, or being bored while paying bills at the table in the kitchen.

The consequences are important too. If the food is "yummy," with lots of fat and calories, it's going to taste good. If there's a good payoff with no negative consequences, the behavior tends to be repeated.

Also, in order to measure change, it's necessary to know the degree, or frequency, of the problem. So you need a system for counting how often it occurs.

Setting Objectives

Once you have a good handle on the problem and know your over-all goal, the next step is to break the problem down into concrete steps or objectives that will achieve that goal. You have actually been learning to do just that, as you have seen how identifying harmful eating habits will effectively help your progress toward your over-all goal of permanent weight management.

Brainstorming Solutions

Once you have decided how you will break down the over-all problem and have specific objectives, you are ready to consider means of achieving them. The best way to approach them is to consider alternative solutions. We call the process brainstorming.

You first try to think of as many different ways as you can for solving the specific objective, say, of stopping extra eating episodes. For example, if paying your bills is accompanied by snacking, then you can avoid this associated behavior by paying them in the bedroom, in the car, taking them to the park, or having your spouse do it. These are all potentially effective solutions to the problem of paying bills in the kitchen where food is stored and snacking occurs.

Deciding on the Best Plan and Trying it Out

Once you have listed all the possible solutions you can think of, then choose the one with the highest probability of success, and get started with it.

Evaluation

Then you judge how successful it is. Was it an effective solution, or an ineffective solution? If you find it effective, make it a habit.

Pat yourself on the back to reinforce the behavior, and if necessary, announce it to the world: "I no longer snack when I'm paying my bills. I put them all in my purse and go down to the park and sit there under the tree with the birds and feel good about myself, away from food—and I pay the damn bills."

Finally, the Reward

Don't forget the reward. There's no fun in solving problems for the intellectual thrill. Make it pay off with a non-caloric reward.

On page 278 I have provided a sample problem solving worksheet, with examples of possible entries. The precise form of the worksheet is not important, but to make full use of this powerful tool, you must go through each step carefully, until you are certain that you have fully explored all possible solutions.

At the end of the lesson you will find a blank Problem Solving Worksheet. Make copies (or make up your own form), and begin using them to attack whatever problems may still stand between you and your over-all weight management goal. When you've solved one problem, don't rest on your laurels, go on to the next one. Be creative and be successful.

SAMPLE PROBLEM SOLVING WORKSHEET

1. OBSERVATION

Possible entry: I seem to eat a lot. (vague)

A better one: I average 12 eating episodes a day.

2. SHORT TERM GOAL SETTING

Possible entry: I'll snack less next week. (not specific)

A better one: I will limit myself to four eating episodes a day.

3. BRAINSTORMING SOLUTIONS

Possible entry: I'll keep track in my mind and use my willpower. (relying on magic)

Another possible entry: I won't allow any food in the house. (unrealistic)

A better one: I will write down everything before I eat it this week.

4. TRYING OUT A SOLUTION

____

(what I did)

5. EVALUATION

Possible entry: If my diary looks o.k. at the end of the week, I'll know I've succeeded. (not concrete enough)

A better one: At the end of the week, I will circle the extra eating episodes I've written in my diary with a red marker.

REWARD

Possible entry: I'll plan my next goal when I accomplish this one. (no reward)

A better one: If I have kept to my plan, I will have my husband take me to a movie next Saturday.

In problem solving, it's necessary to remember to be realistic (make sure you can do it), be specific (general solutions don't work), and to be flexible (don't stick to rigid rules)—if you really are to take charge of your life.

Behavior Modification is Problem Solving

Behavior modification programs are really organized ways of very specifically defining and solving problems. For example, we have defined the problem of eating too rapidly and have offered two solutions: introducing a delay by putting down your fork after each bite; and adding a two-minute delay between courses during the meal.

Up to this point you have been furnished solutions, which you have tried out, but you have not tried to use the separate steps to define and solve a problem. Breaking the problem-solving process into separate steps is very effective, both from the standpoint of first figuring out what to do about the problems, and later potentially to help reanalyze the problems when a solution does not work.

HOMEWORK

As part of the assignment for today, you will compare your eating patterns for last Friday, Saturday, and Sunday with those of Week One. This side-by-side comparison of your beginning habits and those of 17 weeks later should be a good demonstration of how much you have changed.

Transfer the information from your Week One and last week's diaries to the Behavioral Analysis Form included in today's homework section. The fastest way to accomplish this is to ask someone to help you by reading off the columns of items from each food diary. For example, (using the Lesson One Sample Food Diary) under "Minutes Spent Eating," they will read off "10 min., 5 min., 5 min., 1 min., etc." You will add these to get the total time spent eating meals, then divide by the number of meals recorded to get the "average length of meals" for the Behavioral Analysis Form. You will to on to talley totals and averages where called for on the rest of the Behavioral Analysis Form.

Look over your Food Diaries and Behavioral Analysis Form and define a specific small problem. Or, if you do not find one by doing that, think about the topics we have covered that dealt with thoughts and feelings. Ask the person who helped you with the Behavioral Analysis Form to help you look for a specific problem to work on.

Then make a list of all of the possible solutions that come to mind for the *one* specific problem you have selected. Put this problem on your Brainstorming Worksheet. Try to come up with as many creative solutions as you can.

Among the materials for this week is a blank Problem Solving Worksheet, as well as a sample sheet filled out for a hypothetical problem. Make sure you include some method of self-evaluation or feedback with the solution, so you can monitor your progress. This can be a graph, a table, gold stars, or anything that will keep track ofthe behavior you are trying to change. (If you have no way of measuring your problem behavior, you will never know if you are successful.)

Fill out your sheet with the problem and solutions you have chosen. Ask a friend or family member to read it over and help you with solutions to your newly defined eating problem; ask them to witness it by signing on the line labeled "Consultant."

The goal of this exercise is to gain experience and expertise in defining problems and in planning solutions. Make a commitment today to work on definite problems during the coming weeks. In Lesson Nineteen, the first lesson after a brief period of practice and maintenance, you will review your problems, solutions, and successes. If, during the maintenance period you find you have eliminated the problem you define today, define and work on another one. The more the better.

Remember to keep the defined problems very specific. If the problem is one that has already been discussed, for example, eating in one place, and you want to continue working on it for the next weeks, fine. Your observations, defined problems, alternative solutions, ultimate plan, and method of feedback evaluation should all be very clearly spelled out on the Problem Solving Worksheet.

The homework assignment for this week is:

A. Transfer the information from your Lesson One and Lesson Sixteen Food Diaries to your Behavioral Analysis Form. Compare the patterns for these two weeks.

B. Brainstorming Worksheet.

C. Problem solving. Solve at least one problem on the Problem Solving Worksheet.

BEHAVIORAL ANALYSIS FORM—Lesson Seventeen

Sample

	Week 1	Week 16
Number of eating episodes	8	4
Average length of meals	27 mins.	32 mins.
Number of snacks	5	1
Average snack hunger	1	4
Most common body position while eating	3	3
Total time eating at designated eating place	80 mins.	95 mins
Total time only eating while eating	5	90 mins.
"Quality" of food improved—yes/no	—	yes

Which of the behavioral categories has changed most markedly during this 15- week period? ______________________

Can you spot any area that might need further work? ______________

____

BEHAVIORAL ANALYSIS FORM—Lesson Seventeen

	Week 1	Week 16
Number of eating episodes		
Average length of meals		
Number of snacks		
Average snack hunger		
Most common body position while eating		
Total time eating at designated eating place		
Total time only eating while eating		
"Quality" of food improved—yes/no		

Which of the behavioral categories has changed most markedly during this 15- week period? ________________________________

Can you spot any area that might need further work? ____________

____

Remember, no solution is too far out to at least consider.

PROBLEM: ____________________

____

SOLUTION 1: ____________________

____

____

SOLUTION 2: ____________________

____

____

SOLUTION 3: ____________________

____

____

SOLUTION 4: ____________________

____

____

SOLUTION 5: ____________________

____

____

PROBLEM SOLVING WORKSHEET—Lesson Seventeen

1. OBSERVATION

2. SHORT TERM GOAL SETTING

3. BRAINSTORMING SOLUTIONS

4. TRYING OUT A SOLUTION

5. EVALUATION

REWARD

CONSULTANT

LESSON EIGHTEEN MAINTENANCE WEEK #3

WEIGH-IN AND HOMEWORK

Weigh yourself and record the weight and graph your weight change on your Personal Weight Record.

REVIEW

- My total weight loss to date is______.
- Last week I involved my: 1. Spouse 2. Significant Other 3. Child #1, Child #2, Child #3, grandmother, parents (anyone else, including the postman)? Who?____________

For Lesson Seventeen, I discussed the principles of behavioral analysis and problem solving, to get you started toward being your own therapist. In three weeks, this program will end. By then you will be *the expert*. You will be the only one who, six months from now or six years from now, will look at your weight, look at your eating habits, and may say, "I really learned that program," or "Ooops, I better do something!"

Last week I talked about the principles of problem solving in terms of:

1. Observation and long-term goal definition;
2. Identification and definition of specific, well-defined small problems, and short-term goal (or objective) setting;
3. Creative problem solving or brainstorming;
4. Decision making;
5. Feedback and evaluation.

You then used a Problem Solving Worksheet to define a problem, based on observations from your food diaries, to list possible solutions, formulate a plan with some type of feedback, and then to implement your chosen behavioral change program. You compared a weekend from the beginning of your program with a weekend at week seventeen of the program.

Now, looking at your Behavioral Analysis Form, what grade would you give yourself for the change you made during the first 15 weeks of this program? Since we have not discussed many of the individual behaviors for some time, many of the changes you see can be considered new habits. But they still need **PRACTICE** to become life-long habits.

Behavioral analysis and problem solving is one of the keys to maintenance. During the final weeks of this program, you will draw a maintenance weight line which is approximately 3 lbs. above your desired body weight. In the future, if you find that your weight strays above this line, it will be time to start a food diary, sharpen up your behavioral analysis skills, and work on some problem solving techniques.

HOMEWORK

This week is the third and final maintenance session. Review all the lessons up until now, and pick out whichever ones gave you some difficulty.

Lessons reviewed:

1. Introduction to the Behavioral Control of Weight—*Habit Awareness*
2. Home Decalorization—*What You Don't Have You Won't Eat*
3. Cue Elimination—*The Signals that Lead You Astray*
4. Being Active—*The Difference Between Success and Failure*
5. Being Active—*Fitness versus Fatness*
6. Maintenance—*Keys for Survival*
7. Behavior Chains and Alternate Activities—*One Thing Leads to Another*
8. The Act: Eating—*Changing Your Style*
9. Pre-Planning—*Heading Off the Urges*
10. Cue Elimination, Part Two—*Switching More Signals*

11. It's Time to Eat Out—*How to Do It*
12. Maintenance Week—*You Deserve It*
13. How We Think is How We Eat—*Think Before You Buy*
14. Dealing With Feelings—*Think Before You Bite*
15. Stress—*The Soft Underbelly of Fat*
16. Couples—*Is Your Family Fattening?*
17. Behavioral Analysis and Problem Solving—*The Key to Self-Help*

Cross off the title for each lesson you have mastered. If there is any doubt, or if a lesson includes a technique that still needs some sharpening up, circle the lesson title.

If it's something that needs some definite review, write in the words, DO IT! with an exclamation point next to the lesson's name.

During this maintenance week, make up your own food diary if necessary, and use your problem solving techniques to design a problem to work on. If everything's going well, simply fill out the behavioral checklist each day.

Begin today filling out the Daily Behavior Checklist at the end of this lesson, to help yourself keep track of your new behaviors. Read it over each morning before breakfast to remind yourself of the specific techniques we have discussed. In the evening after dinner, rate yourself on a scale of 1-3 on how well you have made use of each of the techniques during the day. This is a subjective measure on your part; there are no right or wrong answers. But consistency in your self-evaluation is important if it is to be meaningful.

During this final maintenance week, practice what you have learned in the first 17 lessons. Carefully weigh yourself each week at the same time of day, and keep your Personal Weight Record and graph up to date. This feedback about your progress is vital to maintaining your program.

This practice period is a time for you to consolidate your learning before you go on to more techniques. Although it is tempting, DO NOT jump ahead to Lesson Nineteen! It would only be asking for failure. You have a whole lifetime to lose weight, and it is important to go about it at a speed that virtually guarantees success. This maintenance will also give you a preview of how hard it will be to continue your new eating skills when there is not the pressure and incentive of a new lesson and new techniques to learn each week.

If you feel like taking extra time for maintenance and practice—DO! There is no gold medal for the first one to finish the book. The rewards are for those who master these techniques.

The homework assignment for this week is:

A. Daily Behavior Checklist

B. Chapter review

C. Technique strengthening

MAINTENANCE WEEK NO. 3

DAILY BEHAVIOR CHECKLIST — Lesson Eighteen

	M	Tu	W	Th	F	Sa	Su
Daily Checklist							
a. reviewed in AM—3 points							
b. reviewed and filled out in the PM— 3 points							
2. Calories stored out of sight (1-3)							
3. Still walking (1-3 — last recorded high mileage = 3, baseline = 0)							
4. Still active whenever possible (1-3)							
5. Preplanning (1 point per meal)							
6. Shopping from a list (1-3)							
7. Taking longer to eat (baseline = 0)							
8. Practice relaxation (5 min = 1, 10 min = 2, 15 min = 3)							
9. Family or other persons involved in my weight loss program (1 = some, 3 = lots)							
10. Less stress related eating (1-3)							

Points Most of the time = 3
Sometimes = 2
Once in a while = 1
No change or not done = 0

Total points for the week ___________

Lesson Eighteen

BEHAVIOR CHECKLIST WEEK 1-18

1. The specific lessons I will review are:

Lesson ______ Title ________________________________

Lesson ______ Title ________________________________

Lesson ______ Title ________________________________

2. The specific technique(s) I will brush up on will be:

________________________________ (Lesson ____)

________________________________ (Lesson ____)

________________________________ (Lesson ____)

LESSON NINETEEN

LIVING IN THE WORLD: PERSONAL GOALS— How to Cope

WEIGH-IN AND HOMEWORK

Weigh yourself and record your weight, and graph your weight change.

My total weight loss for the first 18 weeks is ______.
I am still wasting energy:

- By being more active. Yes ______ No ______
- By increasing my daily mileage. Yes ______ No ______
- By standing when I could be sitting, using the telephone at the other end of the house rather than one closer, parking across the parking lot, and ____________

- Last week I took a shopping list to the market, and stuck to it. Yes ______ No ______
- When I went out to dinner in the last two weeks, I preplanned what I would like to order before I got to the restaurant. Yes ______ No ______
- I asked my spouse—family—parents—loved ones for help last week. Yes ______ No ______

REVIEW

Last week was the final maintenance or practice week of this program. It was a chance to regroup, to look back at all the techniques from the previous lessons, and to do some problem solving. In many ways, the experience of a maintenance week is like the experience of finishing the program, it's a matter of fine tuning, of doing those things that will keep your skills sharp, and keeping the weight that you have lost permanently lost.

PERSONAL GOAL SETTING

As a final part of problem solving, the concept of goal setting and external reinforcement combine to maximize motivation for many people.

We all set goals every day—like "I'll get to work by 8:00 in the morning," or "I'll turn down the dessert at dinner." However, few of us have had training in how to set reasonable goals. Some are too general to be of use in this type of program, like "I'm going to graduate from college"; "I'm going to have a successful career"; or "I'm going to lose weight." Goal setting of this type is not usually very helpful, because it is too vague. The most useful behavior change goals are very specific—for example, "I'm only going to eat three bites of a hamburger for dinner"; or "I'm going to do two push-ups every morning this week."

For personal goals to be useful, it is necessary not only to specify the goal itself, but also the time within which it is to be achieved—It is important to choose goals that are attainable within a definite and fairly short period of time. The chances of success are important too. At least an 80% chance of achieving a goal is desirable, because it gives you a high probability of obtaining the reinforcement that comes with success.

Compare these examples: "I want to lose weight," versus "I want to lose two pounds by a week from today"; or, "I want to be physically fit," versus "I want to be able to run one mile without stopping by the end of the month."

Rewards for reaching specific goals make sense. Compare how you would be motivated by each of the following scenarios: "If I am able to jog one mile a day for five out of seven days, I will receive $100 to spend however I want," versus "As part of my weight control program I should be more active." Which program would be more motivating for you?

The reward need not be great. But it certainly helps when it is there. Be specific: for example, a dollar set aside for each specified achievement, toward a goal of a new dress or tennis racket; or 6 points (out of a hundred needed for tickets to the theatre) for achieving 6 small, immediate objectives; or three hours of baby sitting on Saturday by your husband for achieving a specific goal (for example, eating in one place for 14 consecutive days, or increasing the miles of walking on pedometer records to 30 miles a week).

This week's homework will include a contract establishing rewards for meeting objectives you establish for yourself. It may feel awkward and artificial at first—but it works. After all, isn't the compensation earned for most jobs actually based on the same principle? And isn't changing your eating and exercise patterns work? Perhaps harder work than your job.

JUST SAY NO

We live in a food oriented world. Most entertaining includes food, and most of the out-of-the-office ritual of business includes food. We wine, and dine, and grow overweight. This happens partly because many overweight people have not developed the skill of politely saying no. They are afraid that if they say no, they will offend their host—boss—spouse—mother-in-law—children or—______________ (fill in blank).

This is a matter of simple assertiveness—sticking up for yourself. It's not the same thing as aggressiveness, which can involve pushing people around in an obnoxious and unfeeling way. Looking after your own legitimate needs can be done tactfully, and with a sense of other people's rights and needs—and tends to earn other people's respect.

Assertiveness in our modern world is a survival skill. Assertiveness for the overweight is a weight control skill. It is necessary to go beyond your own feelings and thought processes, and ask people to help you in your weight loss program, even if this means changing the way you interact with people—or even saying NO.

For example, if a husband always brings home candy when he's returning from a business trip, it's all right to suggest that he bring home theatre tickets instead. If birthday parties are traditionally large feasts, it's appropriate to ask that the feast part be toned down, or perhaps another activity be substituted. If that trip to Aunt Minnie's house for Thanksgiving means a six-course meal, and pecan pie, it's okay to thank Aunt Minnie for her good intentions, and at the same time preserve your dietary integrity by taking a small piece, extravagantly praising those few bites, and at the same time explain that you are working on your weight.

Not stating your feelings, or standing up for yourself in eating situations, can be destructive for all concerned. Consider the following scene. George and his wife decide on Saturday night to go out for dinner. They go to a restaurant they haven't been to before (with no preplanning) and look at the menu. George orders a steak with bearnaise sauce (1000 calories). His wife orders Duck a' l'orange (700 calories). The duck comes undercooked. She's unhappy and she mentions to George that she thinks it's a little rare. He tells her that's probably the way it is supposed to be. Since it is a very fancy restaurant and they are polite folks, when the waitress says, "How is everything?" they meekly say, "Just fine."

They both feel tense, and begin to argue—not about the duck or the meal, but about other things, because they are frustrated. The waitress senses something is wrong, stays away from the table, and the service suffers. By dessert, they don't want any (good idea—for the wrong reason). The waitress gets a small tip, George mutters under his breath that he isn't taking his wife here anymore, she tells him in the car that the meal was really terrible. They go home having had a disagreeable evening. They both snack when they get home, and continue to be unhappy with each other. How much easier it would have been had they simply said, "No the duck isn't done to my liking; could you cook it a little bit more?"

The scenario is repeated in restaurants every night, and the tragedy is, no one wins. The restaurant loses business, the waitress gets poor tips, and George and his wife have another unpleasant evening.

Remember, assertiveness is not agressiveness. You don't have to be angry or put people down to assert yourself—you go beyond assertion if you call your wife an idiot because she forgot you were on a diet and baked you a cake for your birthday; or loudly call for the manager because of the undercooked duck, rather than letting the waitress handle it.

Assertiveness is asking for what you want, in a polite but firm manner. When the waiter brings bread, it's all right to say, "I don't care for any," or "Please take it back to the kitchen." No explanation is needed. When the waiter asks what salad dressing you would like, it is acceptable to ask for it on the side, or to ask whether diet dressing is available.

When you are unsure how food will be cooked at a restaurant, rather than wait to dissect it after it reaches the table, you can ask how the food is prepared before you order—often this will be seen as a compliment (and be cordially received). And it's a good way to make sure there aren't hidden fats in the food.

This principle applies to countless other situations. Just because you think no one else seems to exercise, you don't have to stay inside your hotel room when you are in Manhattan. Brave the crowds, brave the looks, and go for a run in the park (but not at night—there's bravery and there's stupidity). At home, if you feel you are not getting the support you need, ask for it. One need not be accusing in order to say, "Please help me." Remember, it is your *right* to control your social environment.

HOMEWORK

The homework for this week is very simple.

There is an Assertive Behavior Summary for the week. The type of entries you might make would include asking the waiter to take the bread back to the kitchen, politely declining to have a dessert, requesting that the salad dressing be given to you on the side, asking your family to have a low-calorie entree, or even asking someone to go for a walk with you after dinner.

Write down each time that you did one of these things, and the outcome. Did everyone hate you? Was it a great disappointment to everyone? Did Aunt Minnie disown you? Did you get thrown out of the restaurant? Did you get laughed at or humiliated? Did your spouse threaten to leave you? Probably not. The chances are overwhelming that people respected your requests and complimented you on your good judgment, and that you avoided a few extra calories.

Secondly, there is a Contingency Contract to fill out with someone close to you. Specify what behavior you are going to change this coming week—and what the reward will be! You'll be surprised at how this can help your motivation.

The homework assignment for this week is:

A. Assertive Behavior Summary

B. Contingency Contract

Lesson Nineteen

ASSERTIVE BEHAVIOR SUMMARY

Examples of assertive behavior (choose one each day)

	Outcome
Monday	
Tuesday	
Wednesday	
Thursday	
Friday	
Saturday	
Sunday	

Lesson Nineteen

CONTINGENCY CONTRACT

1. My goal for this week is to ______________________________

____

2. To achieve this, I will ______________________________

____

____

3. I will keep track of my progress by ______________________________

____

____

4. My reward for achieving this will be ______________________________

____

____

5. ______________________________ (person) will give me my reward on

______________________________ (day) after they review my progress.

signed ______________________________ (you)

signed ______________________________ (witness)

LESSON TWENTY

SNACKS, CUES, AND HOLIDAYS— How to Celebrate

WEIGH-IN AND HOMEWORK

Weigh yourself and record and graph your weight on your Personal Weight Record.

Last week you continued the review of your progress, and learned about personal goal setting, contingency contracting, and the need for standing up to "food-bearers" and others.

- How did you feel about the contingency contracting?
- Did it help motivate you to reach some specific behavioral goal?
  Yes ______ No ______
- Was the reward you picked worth the task you had to complete?
  Yes ______ No ______
- Was the behavioral goal simple enough to be achievable?
  Yes ______ No ______

REVIEW

Specific goal setting—and specific rewards—are the keys to this type of external motivation. Contingency contracting can be one of the most powerful techniques available to you for weight loss maintenance. A contract with a loved one or even a fellow employee, to achieve specific behavioral goals over the next six months (taken a week or two at a time), will help insure that you keep your end of the bargain—and change.

- Were you successful in asserting yourself? How many times for the week? ______

- At home? Yes ______ No ______

- At work? Yes ______ No ______

- Other ______ Yes ______ No ______

Assertiveness skills in eating situations are as vital as preplanning, choosing low-caloric density foods, not responding to environmental stimuli that provoke snacking, and increasing your activity. If you allow others to abuse or love you with food, they will make you fat. Don't let them get away with it.

DEALING WITH HOLIDAYS

Holidays are times of particular difficulty with food. In all cultures around the world, holidays are accompanied by feasting. Whether it's Thanksgiving, Christmas, a birthday, or the Fourth of July picnic, traditionally we accompany it with food. Unfortunately, the main course is rarely carrot sticks. Aunt Minnie arrives with that wonderful chicken liver paté, a triple layer chocolate cake, or Grandmother's recipe for candied yams with marshmallow and brandy sauce—as well as Uncle George and the punch. There's every type of delectable food known to mankind, and it's hard to say no.

That's the bad news. The good news is that feasts are predictable. You know your family, you know your festivities, you know your feasts, and you know how to say no. It need not be a shock each time.

Think ahead for Thanksgiving dinner. It could very easily be a 6,000-calorie bash. You don't have to stand out like a sore thumb to say no—what can you do to limit the number of calories you consume, leaving others to devour yams with brandy sauce?

Think back to Lesson Nine. You learned to plan ahead to have smaller portions, to eliminate some food items. We'll work with those techniques as applied to special occasions, as part of our homework for this week.

Some of what was covered last week can help too. In Lesson Nineteen, you learned to say no with a smile. Your new assertiveness may enable you even to suggest a change in the traditional menu.

What about the standard feast they prepare for you on your birthday? How about a suggestion for theatre tickets instead?

Remember, you needn't suffer in silence, or even suffer. You live in a social environment, and you've already asked them for their help. Your family can even plan together to change their feasting style, and add other activities to the family get-togethers.

Even the desserts can be pared of some of their calories. Think ahead about what would taste good at the end of a meal; there are some wonderful treats with a lot less calories than french apple pie with ice cream.

NEW TOPIC: SNACK CONTROL (EATING WITH INFORMED CONSENT)

Snacks are usually eaten in response to psychological, not physiological hunger. The hunger pangs that lead to snacking are almost always triggered by environmental stimuli. These hunger cues are situation specific and time limited, usually lasting about 20 minutes. In other words, if you move away from the situation, or don't respond to the cues by eating, the feeling of hunger will go away.

For example, imagine yourself walking down the street on a sunny morning, thinking about the coming weekend with a day off from work. Suddenly, you pass a bakery shop. The sight of fresh pastries in the window and the smell from the open door are very powerful cues. They cause you to react with a sensation of hunger—even though ten seconds before you had no thoughts of food or hunger.

If you remove yourself rapidly from the situation, the hunger will fade away. Or, if you don't leave, but stand in front of the shop in the presence of the cues long enough without responding to them (by eating), the hunger will also go away. However, if you go in and have a fresh doughnut, the urge to snack will be even stronger next time.

Snacking may not be a problem for you at this point. However, there are two situations where it may reemerge. The first is during vacations or holidays, where the environment is saturated with food. The second is the snacking that occurs in the context of an ordinary meal. There is no difference between eating that larger dessert or third piece of chicken now, "because it is on the table," and having it as a snack later, "because it is in the refrigerator."

Only eat what you need—leave the rest on the table. If you can control the impulse to eat when you are not hungry, you will dramatically decrease your caloric intake without depriving yourself or feeling hungry.

As I have discussed, hunger pangs usually are induced by stimuli in your environment. One type of example was given above, where you feel a pang of hunger when you suddenly see some attractive food, even though you were not thinking about eating. Another type of cue is found in chains of associations that lead to eating.

To give one example of an association chain: On a Sunday drive, you see a perfectly shaped pine tree which reminds you of Christmas, which recalls the memory of childhood Christmases and the turkey dinner that mother used to make, which in turn makes you feel hungry. If you weren't aware of this progression of associations, you might pull over at the next Howard Johnson's. But if you recognize the cause of your hunger, you have a chance of combatting it effectively.

You have learned a great number of snack inhibiting techniques in the past 19 lessons, some of which will be appropriate to almost any situation. Although they were introduced in different contexts, they will be your first line of defense during holidays and vacations. With some reflection you will see how to apply them to impulse eating in any situation.

The techniques most commonly used to combat impulses are:

1. Introduce an eating delay. Set a timer when you feel hungry, and have your snack only after you have waited a predetermined amount of time. Progressively increase the length of time before your snack.
2. If you snack, put the food down between bites, take longer to eat the snack, and enjoy the food. If you permit yourself to do this, you won't feel guilty about eating, and you will tend to eat less over a longer period of time.
3. Snack only at your Designated Appropriate Eating Place.
4. Substitute alternate activities for eating. Either modify the behavior chain that leads to eating, while the impulse is still remote from food, or, when you are actually confronted with the snack, substitute an incompatible behavior or a low-calorie snack food.
5. Pre-plan your food intake to decrease the strength of your impulses.
6. Only buy foods on a full stomach, and avoid buying snack foods for future use.
7. Leave some behind—part of a cookie, a piece of popcorn, a bit of cake. When you are finished, throw it away.

In other words, control your environment. Don't let it control you!

How Do You Feel About Your Progress with These Techniques?

- Do you remember the cue elimination techniques just mentioned?
  Yes ______ No ______
- Are you still using them every day?
  Yes ______ No ______
- Which ones are most useful for your snacks?

  1. ______________________________
  2. ______________________________
  3. ______________________________
- Do you feel that you are beginning to control your environment?
  Yes ______ No ______

You are about to receive some new techniques for your snack prevention program. However, in order to make sense out of them, you need to know more about the physiology of eating and hunger.

Several investigators have made basic observations about the biology of hunger that bear directly on impulse eating. (9) They asked individuals who had gone without food for a standard amount of time to drink an entire meal of chocolate liquid through a straw. The subjects could not see into the food container, and they had no external way of knowing how much liquid they were consuming. In addition, they did not know the calorie content of the drink; it could be (and was) varied as much as tenfold before the subjects could taste the difference. In the experiment the liquid always looked, felt, and tasted the same. They simply drank the chocolate-flavored liquid until they felt full.

The results of the experiments were surprising. One psychologist found that subjects drank the same amount of fluid every day, despite marked changes in caloric content. Volume or bulk appeared to be the factor that told people when they were satisfied.

Another psychologist found that belief is a critical variable in the subjective feeling of being full. If subjects believed a liquid meal was high in calories, they were satisfied with less than if they believed it was low in calories. Like the other study, the actual caloric content of the food was irrelevant.

The conclusions were: *Over the short term, humans cannot sense the caloric content of food.* People only began to "feel" hunger after they had been on a low-calorie liquid for several days.

These experiments appear to contradict many current ideas about hunger—for example, the notion that hunger is satisfied by raising your blood sugar. At the present time no one knows how the brain senses "fullness." Volume, and *belief* in calorie content are not the entire answer, but they are important.

We can make use of the volume sensors in several ways. When you have an overwhelming urge for a snack, make sure it has volume. Precede each snack with a large glass of water, a diet drink, or some food with volume (like Bran) and few calories. If it is a conditioned and not a physiological hunger, this will help you ignore the pangs. Eventually, whatever is telling you to be hungry will begin to lose its power over you—it will no longer be rewarded with food.

Do You Understand This?

- Can you define hunger?
  Yes ______ No ______

- Describe where you feel hunger and what it feels like.

  ____

  ____

  ____

- Did you understand the hunger and volume experiments?
  Yes ______ No ______

- Do you see how bulk can help decrease your hunger sensations?
  Yes ______ No ______

The volume experiments also suggest a strategy for controlling meals. Include some bulk, whether liquid or solid (like a large salad), before you eat your main course. This will provide the internal sensation of satiety sooner than if you eat in the reverse order.

The technique of incorporating bulk in your diet *must* be used in conjunction with the techniques we introduced previously. There is no reason to inhibit your hunger response unless you are developing the habit of eating only in response to hunger. To put it another way, there is little point in working on your hunger by eating your salad first, if you still feel compelled to eat everything on your plate, or if you still eat everything because your attention is drawn away by another activity like reading.

A second technique for snacking is food substitution: using low-calorie foods for snacks. Sometimes you will crave caviar. When that happens, you should have it and enjoy it. Don't worry about the calories. At other times, you may be satisfied with something low in calories.

Part of your decision will be based on how many calories you think there are in foods available to you. If you are given a choice between duck and lobster at a fancy party, there is no intuitive way to know what the caloric content of each is. If you are tired of duck, you might choose lobster by chance for variety. However, if you know that there are only 95 calories in 3-1/2 ounces of lobster, you might decide to save 250 calories by having it instead of the same amount of duck.

HOMEWORK

Since the caloric content of foods is often not obvious, effective snack substitution depends on knowledge about caloric content. We have included some snack hints with today's materials, to help you look at the caloric content of impulse foods and to help you at critical points—when you are at a party, buffet, reception, or looking for something to nibble on at home. Knowledge about the relative numbers of calories will help you make your decisions. This information will be most helpful when there are equally tempting choices.

After Lesson Five you were asked to acquire a simple calorie counter. Your task now is to: (1) make a list of your favorite snacks on the Snack Worksheet in the homework materials for this week; (2) choose an alternate snack from the calorie book; (3) figure out your savings by subtracting the calories in the substitute snack from the calories in the original snack.

Then, to make this calculation really meaningful, figure how much this daily caloric saving would mean in terms of pounds over a full year. (Simply multiply the daily saving of calories by 365, the number of days in a year, and divide the result by 3500, the number of calories in a pound of fat.)

Finally: The best anti-snack technique of all! In Lesson Seven you learned about food urges—and ways of combatting them by substituting alternate activities. Ask yourself before each snack episode—"Am I hungry, or just snacking?" If the answer is "I'm just snacking," then stop and do something else!

Are There Still Some Questions?

- Do you still have questions about how to use bulk to combat hunger?
  Yes ______ No ______
  (Although it may not be effective all of the time, it will be effective enough of the time to help you cut down on your total intake.)

- Do you see how this technique could be used before a party?
  Yes ______ No ______

- Do you see how some knowledge of snack calories fits into this program?
  Yes ______ No ______

- Do you understand how to use the Snack Worksheet?
  Yes ______ No ______

You have learned many techniques which can help you deal with snacks. They may not be as relevant at the present time as they will be during a vacation or holiday. Remember, however, that these techniques are easier to practice now. Later you will be confronted with an overwhelming array of foods, hors d'oeuvres, and birthday and Christmas goodies, and it will be much harder to remember your new coping skills at the height of temptation if you don't practice now—at a time of lower temptation.

Finally, on the Special Occasion Meal Planner form in the homework for this week, plan a menu for Thanksgiving. Write down the hors d'oeuvres, entree, drinks, and dessert. See how few calories you can put into the meal, and still retain the festive atmosphere—and fun with good food! Include plans for the way it's arranged on the plate, the way it's served, the table decorations, and other festivities.

Then try the same type of menu planning for a birthday celebration. In addition to celebrating someone being one year older, you're also celebrating being quite a few pounds thinner yourself. Then go on to plan another feast day—as many as you can think of.

The homework for this week is:

A. Keep track of your activity on the Daily Activity Record.

B. Fill in the Snack Worksheet.

C. Fill in the Special Occasions Meal Planner.

DAILY ACTIVITY RECORD

(Fill in miles per day walked and minutes of exercise or extra activities)

	Monday		Tuesday		Wednesday		Thursday		Friday		Saturday		Sunday	
	Miles	Calories	Miles	Calories	Miles	Calories	Miles	Calories	Miles	Calories	Miles	Calories	Miles	Calories
Miles Walked														
Activity or Exercise	Mins.	Calories	Mins.	Calories	Mins.	Calories	Mins.	Calories	Mins.	Calories	Mins.	Calories	Mins.	Calories

Use the table on page 109 and 110 to calculate the caloric equivalent of each activity. If your activity is not included, chose one from the list that is similar.

Lesson Twenty

SNACK HINTS

1. Make snacks hard to get. They should require preparation, like popcorn, or be hard to eat, like frozen bananas.
2. Try to avoid extremes of intake—neither starvation nor overeating. They both lead to feast/famine cycles, and extra eating between meals. Never skip a meal if you're hungry—eat with control.
3. High protein food will decrease food cravings—they last longer.

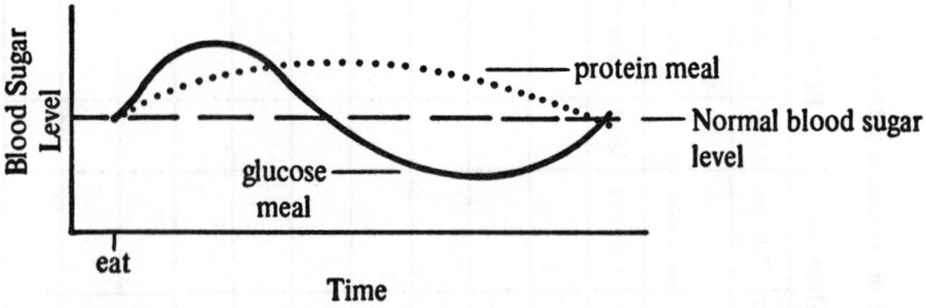

4. A small glass of unsweetened fruit juice will help you overcome that famished feeling—combine it with a high protein snack if necessary.
5. Tea and coffee (even decaffeinated) stimulate stomach secretions and hunger.
6. Alcohol is caloric, stimulates hunger, and leads to higher levels of blood triglycerides.
7. Read labels. Some artificial creamers use coconut (saturated fat) oil instead of corn oil and may contain more calories. Diet colas vary from nearly 0 to 35 per can. Water-packed foods have many fewer calories than syrup-packed. The order in which the contents are listed indicate how much of each is present inside the container. For example-the Cheerios label says it contains oat flower, wheat starch, sugar, salt, sodium phosphate. Sugar is the third most prevalent constituent of Cheerios.
8. Carry a low-calorie sweetner with you.
9. If quantity is your weakness, add bulk; for example, raw vegetables, long grain rice, a diet soda before dinner, or starting dinner with boullion for a soup course.
10. Keep in mind that one mixed drink like a margarita is roughly calorically equal to a Hershey Bar, or a cream-filled cupcake.
11. Try to always have an alternate response to snack eating—keep in mind, a little hunger is the feeling of losing weight.

SNACK WORKSHEET

SAMPLE

	For This Food	Substitute	Savings
EXAMPLE.	CAVIAR, 3.5 OZ. – 316 CAL.	CRAB MEAT, 3.5 OZ 93 CAL.	223 CAL.
	DUCK, 3.5 OZ. – 350 CAL.	LOBSTER MEAT, 3.5 OZ 95 CAL.	255 CAL.
	BEER-(SCHLITZ, 12 OZ) 150 CAL	BEER (MILLER LITE) 12 OZ 96 CAL	54 CAL.
	HOSTESS TWINKIE 144 CAL	2-SUNSHINE FIG BARS 90 CAL	54 CAL.

SNACK WORKSHEET

For This Food	Substitute	Savings

SPECIAL OCCASION MEAL PLANNER-Lesson Twenty

Thanksgiving Menu

	Calories per serving
Hor d'oeuvres	______
Entree	______
Salad	______
Drinks	______
Dessert	______
Total	______

Notes on table decorations,
food arrangements, etc.:

Birthday Menu

	Calories per serving
Hor d'oeuvres	______
Entree	______
Salad	______
Drinks	______
Dessert	______
Total	______

Notes on table decorations,
food arrangements, etc.:

Other Feast Day

	Calories per serving
Hor d'oeuvres	______
Entree	______
Salad	______
Drinks	______
Dessert	______
Total	______

Notes on table decorations,
food arrangements, etc.:

LESSON TWENTY-ONE

THE END AND BEGINNING—

Here's to a New Life—and Lifestyle

WEIGH-IN AND HOMEWORK

Weigh yourself and record and graph your weight on your Personal Weight Record.

- I have lost ______ lbs. in the past 20 weeks.
- How many miles did you record on your pedometer last week? ______
- How does that compare with your baseline that you measured week 2? ______

REVIEW: SNACKS, CUES, AND HOLIDAYS (EATING WITH INFORMED CONSENT)

Last week you reviewed many of the techniques introduced during the first eight lessons to control impulse eating or snacking. These techniques are successful because hunger pangs are usually a reflex response to external cues. They are usually not related to a physiological need for food.

These impulses to eat are time limited; if you do not respond to them, they will go away. Every time you are able to "wait out" an impulse to eat, the cue will become weaker. Each time that particular cue occurs and is not rewarded with food, its strength will decrease and it will provoke a reduced hunger response, until it eventually becomes neutral. You are probably aware at this point of several environmental cues, like television, that have become more neutral—they no longer provoke hunger, or at the least lead to much less desire for a snack.

Although snacks are under fairly good control for most people at this point in the program, there is a tendency for snacking to reemerge during holidays and vacations, when the environment is saturated with food cues and large meals, and when pleasure is the order of the day.

These meals often include a snack added to a regular meal. You can recognize it by the rationalizations that allow you to eat a little bit more than you really need—for example, an extra piece of chicken "because it is there on the table," or a large piece of cake "because someone has to eat it," or hors d'oeuvres "because they were offered to me." Many times you can counteract the urge to snack by simply asking yourself the question, "Am I hungry?" If the answer is "no" (if your hunger rating scale would show 0, 1, or 2), then you should try to pass up the food.

The two new concepts introduced last week were: first, the use of bulk, e.g., a salad or a glass or water, to provide the sensation of satiety earlier in a meal or snack, and second, the use of caloric information. You need to know the calorie content of foods so you can make an informed decision about what to eat. You bought a calorie counter and used it with the Snack Worksheet to give yourself some information about impulse foods.

The caloric content of foods is not intuitively obvious, and this is especially true of snack foods (one ounce of Triskets® has 120 calories; an ounce of Rye Krisp® 90; an ounce of potato chips 150)—which usually are presented in a situation where you have choices. If you know the caloric content of the foods you are offered, it is easy to choose the one with fewer calories. For now, the only calories you should be counting are those needed to do the homework, and those in snacks. The latter are important because we want you to be able to make conscious informed choices between foods.

How Have You Been Doing?

- Did you look up the caloric value of your snack foods?
  Yes ______ No ______

- Were you able to substitute snack foods and save calories?
  Yes ______ No ______

- Were you able to use bulk to decrease your hunger?
  Yes ______ No ______

- What kinds of bulk did you use?

  1. ______________________________

  2. ______________________________

  3. ______________________________

You've had an introduction to the behavioral techniques effective for weight loss maintenance. In 20 weeks, however, you can only begin to experiment with behavioral self-control.

As you have found out, eating is not a simple matter. It is intimately associated with every aspect of your life, from relationships to nutrition, to activity, to assertiveness. The only way to make what you have learned permanent is to practice. The only way habits die is by conscious avoidance and by substituting new, more healthy, and creative habits.

I want you to continue to monitor the world around you. Your weight loss program isn't over, even though you have finished this book. Next week, and every week after that, continue to pat yourself on the back when you're successful. Buy yourself gifts to celebrate your successes. When you are able to keep the fat out of your house, compliment yourself and your family. When you're able to deal with emotions without eating, reflect on how far you've come, and what a good job you're doing.

On the other hand, when you feel like you've blown it, simply recognize that you're human, and that you can pick up the pieces and keep on going. The worst thing is to begin negative self-talk, and tell yourself that since you've blown it, you might as well blow it all away—that you're destined to be fat.

SUMMARY

Maintenance is much easier if you have strong environmental support from your family and friends. In this program you have learned some of the ground rules for establishing that support. If you shared today's lesson with the people who make up your social environment, then you have greatly increased your chances of maintaining your behavior changes and weight loss.

The one homework form you will probably want to keep using regularly is a Maintenance Behavior Checklist. The most effective way of using the Maintenance Behavior Checklist is as a "cue card" for feedback and evaluation. Read it before each meal, and record your performance at the end of the day.

If you want to analyze your eating behaviors, either now or in the future, keep a detailed food diary for one week. Make up a food diary form that includes your problem areas, or copy one from this book. When it is filled out, you will have a good picture of how well your behaviors are being maintained, and what areas need improvement.

MAINTENANCE TRAINING PROGRAM

Although you are at the end of this book, you have really only started your weight control program. Like graduating from college, now the real work starts. You have tools in the areas of dietary management, physical activity, behaviorial change, psychological adjustment, and environmental control to create a new, more active lifestyle with more controlled eating. The key to maintenance and continued weight loss is *self-observation.* Keep using the materials presented to you.

Long-term success in weight control programs can be predicted for those who:

- eat in a controlled style
- continue to exercise
- are more active physically
- eat less calorically dense foods
- assert themselves in eating situations
- have the support of those around them
- think differently about food, appetite, and hunger than they did when they were overweight
- free themselves from environmental cues to eat
- do not eat for emotional reasons
- can problem solve to eliminate extra eating
- contract with themselves and others to achieve short and long-term goals

- enjoy being thinner
- take on the responsibility for monitoring their eating behaviors and their weight long after they have achieved a normal body weight

As a first step, continue to keep a weekly weight graph. Select a regular day of the week for your weigh-in. Each morning, on that day of the week, weigh yourself with no clothes on. Enter this weight on your Personal Weight Record.

Once you have achieved your desired body weight, don't stop. On your weight graph, draw a line with a red pencil three pounds above your desired body weight. If your weight goes above this line, immediately resume your weight control program: increase your activity, and do some problem solving. Something will have gone wrong. But not hopelessly wrong. Define the problem with a food diary if necessary, and devise a behavioral change program. Get your weight back under the red line!

A guaranteed step toward failure is to feel defeated, and then to put off any effort at correction for a few more pounds—to refuse to work on the problem because you "blew it." (A few pounds after that, you will give up altogether.) Don't be afraid to be human. Correct yourself as soon as you've made an error.

You've had an introduction to the behavioral techniques for weight loss and weight loss maintenance. In the twenty weeks of this program you have only begun to experiment with behavioral self-control. *Practice*. The only way new behaviors become habits is by practice and endless repetition. The only way to make old habits die is by not repeating them, and to substitute new, more healthy, adaptive, creative ways of living.

Continue to monitor the world around you, and your own attitudes. When you're successful at losing weight, increasing activity, or changing a behavior, pat yourself on the back, or even buy yourself a gift.

Pay attention to your improved health status. It is well worth working for, even though it is one of the last rewards of weight loss that you may become aware of. It may mean years of additional illness-free life for you.

When you are eating less calorically dense food, make it a habit to keep high-calorie foods out of the house, and away from your work. Even go so far as to be assertive and tell others you don't want to be around it—that you are freed from the world of Twinkies and fudge—and that you want to stay free.

When you're able to deal with your emotions without eating, to express your feelings, and not run for the refrigerator, reflect on how far you've come, and what a good job you're doing.

PAYBACK—THE CONTINGENT REFUND TO YOURSELF

It is time for you to reward yourself for completing the homework in the course. Each assignment had a cash value. Although it has not been a great deal of money for each assignment, cumulatively it has added up to an amount you may care about. The return of the money you have earned is a good way of showing yourself how well you have done in the program.

Add up the amount of money you have earned on your Homework Credit Sheet. Take the amount you did not earn and give it away—to your children, your spouse, or to a charity. Put the rest of the money in your pocket—it is yours! Do with it whatever you want. Don't spend it on something for someone else. Don't put it back in the family kitty. You earned it—you spend it.

MAINTENANCE BEHAVIOR CHECKLIST

Weeks 21-40	21	22	23	24	25	26	27	28	29	30	31	32	33	34	35	36	37	38	39	40
1. Behavior checklist completed																				
2. Aware of / not responding to food cues																				
3. Continued exercise/walking																				
4. Continued extra activity																				
5. In control of eating situations/assertive																				
6. Less "emotional eating"																				
7. Preplanning meals/shopping																				
8. Family support asked for/received																				
9. "Thinner" attitudes towards food appetite and self image																				
10. Eating less calorically dense food																				
Week Total																				

Pick one day a week to weigh yourself, and to fill in the maintenance behavior check list. Rate each item on a scale of 1 (better than when you started) to 3 (done most of the time). If your total score begins to drop during the next 19 weeks, do some problem solving. Make a copy of this checklist so you can keep practicing your "thin" behaviors for the coming year—by then they should be permanent.

APPENDIX

Sample

Personal Weight Record

Name F.S.
Date 7-18 Height 5'9"

Date	Weight	Weight Change	Total Wt. Change
7-18	236¼	—	—
7-25	233	-3¼	-3¼
8-1	228½	-4½	-7¾
8-8	228¼	-¼	-8
8-15	225¾	-2½	-10½
8-22	223	-2¾	-13¼
8-29	221	-2	-15¼
9-5	219	-2	-17¼
9-12	221	+2	-15¼
9-19	219	-2	-17¼
9-26	219	0	-17¼
10-3	214½	-4½	-21¾
10-10	217½	+3	-18¾
10-17	214	-3½	-22¼
10-24	213	-1	-23¼
10-31	vacation		
11-7	214½	+1½	-21¾
11-14	218	+3½	-18¼
11-21	214	-4	-22¼
11-28	Thanksgiving Vacation		

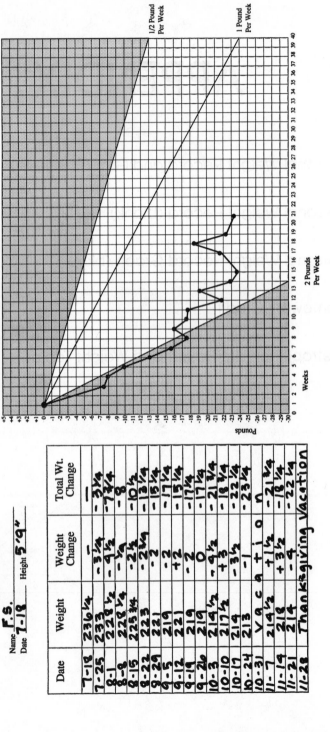

Personal Weight Record - Graph

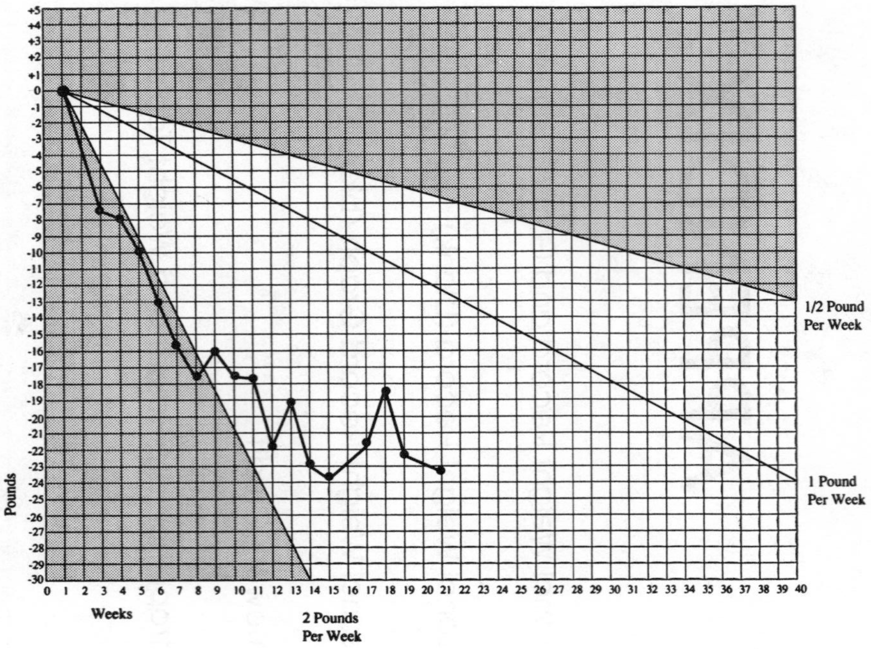

Personal Weight Record

Name ______________________________

Date ___________ Height ___________

Date	Weight	Weight Change	Total Wt. Change

APPENDIX

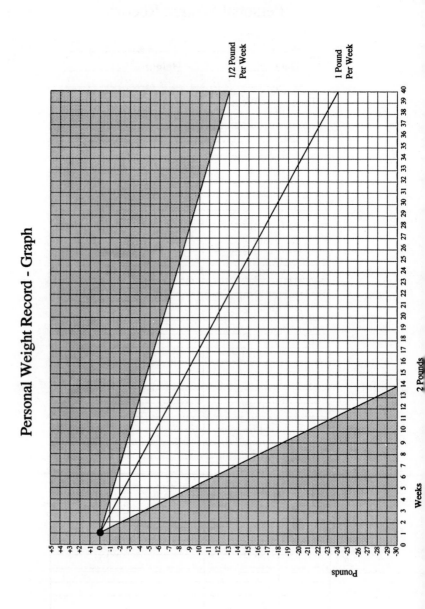

Personal Weight Record - Graph

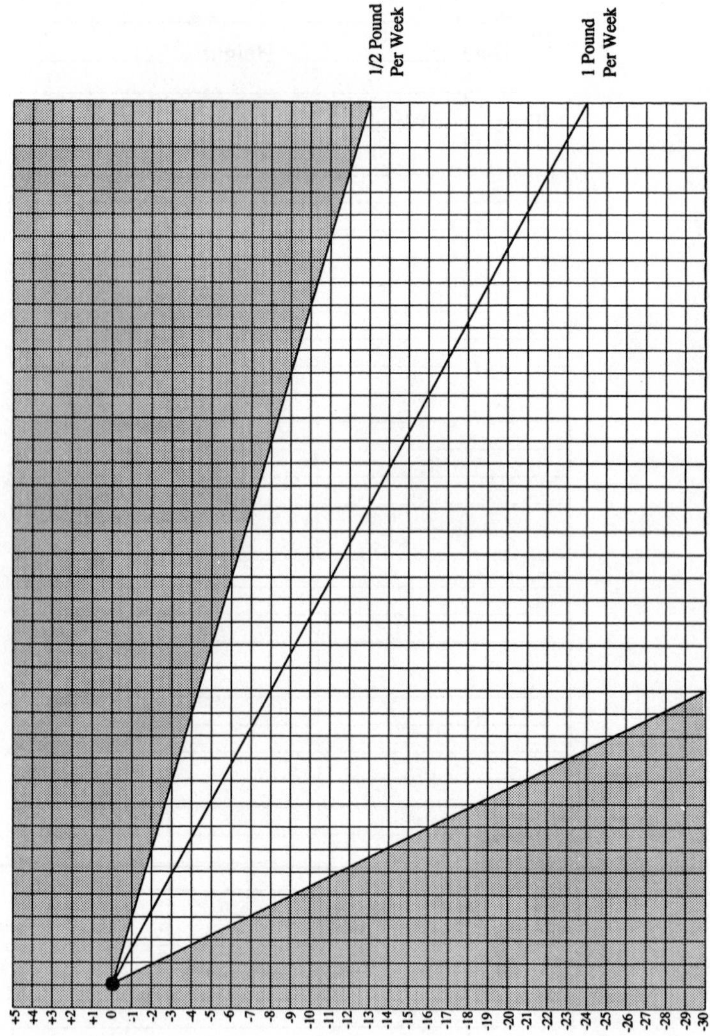

APPENDIX-HOMEWORK CREDIT

		done	value	due me
Lesson 1	**Introduction / Habit Awareness**			
	Food diary		3.00	
	Eating episode location		1.00	
	Food storage location		1.00	
Lesson 2	**Home Decalorization**			
	Food diary		2.50	
	Remove food to kitchen/storage		2.50	
Lesson 3	**Cue Elimination**			
	Food diary		1.50	
	Eat at designated place		.50	
	Change places		.50	
	Only eat		.50	
	Opaque containers		.50	
	Junk food out of sight		.50	
	Serving dishes off the table		.50	
	Eating place record		.50	
Lesson 4	**Being Active**			
	Food diary		1.50	
	Food out of sight		1.00	
	Daily activity record		1.50	
	Eating place record		1.00	
Lesson 5	**Being Active**			
	Food diary		2.00	
	Daily activity record		1.00	
	Daily energy out (activity) graph		1.00	
	Eating place record		1.00	
Lesson 6	**Maintenance**			
	Daily behavior checklist		2.50	
	Daily activity record		2.50	
Lesson 7	**Behavior Chains/ Alternate Activities**			
	Food/activity diary		1.00	
	Alternate activity sheet		2.00	
	Behavior"unlinking" strategy		2.00	
Lesson 8	**The Act of Eating**			
	Food diary		2.50	
	Daily activity record		2.50	
Lesson 9	**Preplanning**			
	Shopper's helper reviewed		1.00	
	Daily behavior checklist		1.00	
	Daily activity sheet		1.00	
	Food diary (preplanning worksheet)		2.00	

Lesson l0	**Cue Elimination Part Two**			
	Daily behavior checklist		2.50	
	Food diary		2.50	
Lesson 11	**It's Time to Eat Out**			
	Menu preparation		2.50	
	Daily activity record		2.50	
Lesson 12	**Practice**			
	Behavior change list		5.00	
Lesson 13	**How We Think is How We Eat**			
	Food diary		2.50	
	Daily activity record		2.50	
Lesson 14	**Dealing with Feelings**			
	Mileage record		1.00	
	Script writing		2.00	
	Urge-snack-feelings,and behaviors		2.00	
Lesson 15	**Stress**			
	Urge-snack-feelings, and behaviors		1.00	
	Script writing		2.00	
	Stress monitoring record		2.00	
Lesson 16	**Couples**			
	Stress monitoring record		1.00	
	Cooperation checklist		2.00	
	Food diary		2.00	
Lesson 17	**Behavioral Analysis and Problem Solving**			
	Behavioral analysis form		2.00	
	Brainstorming worksheet		1.50	
	Problem solving		1.50	
Lesson 18	**Maintaince No. 3**			
	Behavior checklist		2.00	
	Chapter review		1.50	
	Technique strengthening		1.50	
Lesson 19	**Living in the World**			
	Assertive behavior summary		3.00	
	Contingency contract		2.00	
Lesson 20	**Snacks-Cues-Holidays**			
	Daily activity record		2.00	
	Snack worksheet		1.50	
	Special occasion meal planner		1.50	
Total			$100.00	$

1983 Metropolitan Height & Weight Tables

Weights at ages 25-59 based on lowest mortality. Weight in pounds according to frame (in indoor clothing weighing 5 lbs for men and 3 lbs for women; shoes with 1" heels. Courtesy of Metropolitan Life Insurance Company.

MEN

Height Feet	Inches	Small Frame	Medium Frame	Large Frame
5	2	128-134	131-141	138-150
5	3	130-136	133-143	140-153
5	4	132-138	135-145	142-156
5	5	134-140	137-148	144-160
5	6	136-142	139-151	146-164
5	7	138-145	142-154	149-168
5	8	140-148	145-157	152-172
5	9	142-151	148-160	155-176
5	10	144-154	151-163	158-180
5	11	146-157	154-166	161-184
6	0	149-160	157-170	164-188
6	1	152-164	160-174	168-192
6	2	155-168	164-178	172-197
6	3	158-172	167-182	176-202
6	4	162-176	171-187	181-207

WOMEN

Height Feet	Inches	Small Frame	Medium Frame	Large Frame
4	10	102-111	109-121	118-131
4	11	103-113	111-123	120-134
5	0	104-115	113-126	122-137
5	1	106-118	115-129	125-140
5	2	108-121	118-132	128-143
5	3	111-124	121-135	131-147
5	4	114-127	124-138	134-151
5	5	117-130	127-141	137-155
5	6	120-133	130-144	140-159
5	7	123-136	133-147	143-163
5	8	126-139	136-150	146-167
5	9	129-142	139-153	149-170
5	10	132-145	142-156	152-173
5	11	135-148	145-159	155-176
6	0	138-151	148-162	158-179

REFERENCES

1. Stunkard, A.J., New Therapies for the Eating Disorders: Behavior Modification of Obesity and Anorexia Nervosa, *Arch. Gen. Psych., 26:*391-398, 1972.

2. Schacter, S., and Rodin, J., *Obese Humans and Rats*, Lawrence Erlbaum Associates, Potomac, Maryland, 1974.

3. Schacter, S., and Gross, L.P., Manipulated Time and Eating Behaviors, *Journal of Personality and Social Psychology, 10:*98-106, 1968.

4. Stewart, S., and David, B., *Slim Chance in a Fat World*, Research Press, Champaign, Illinois, 1972, p. 85.

5. Mayer, J., and Bullen, B., Nutrition and Athletic Performance, *Physiological Reviews, 40:*369-397, 1960.

6. Margen, S., Energy Balance with Increasing Weight, in Wilson, N.L. (ed), *Obesity*, F.A. Davis, Philadelphia, 1969, pp. 77-89.

7. Mayer, J., *Overweight: Causes, Costs, and Control*, Prentice Hall, Englewood Cliffs, New Jersey, 1969, pp. 69-83.

8. Mayer, J., *Overweight: Causes, Costs, and Control*, Prentice Hall, Englewood Cliffs, New Jersey, 1969, pp. 79.

9. Wooley, S.C., Physiologic versus Cognitive Factors in Short-Term Food Regulation in the Obese and Nonobese, *Psychosomatic Medicine, 34:* 62-68, 1972.

BIBLIOGRAPHY

The individual techniques in this manual have been collected from many sources. In most cases, it is impossible to say who first thought of each individual therapeutic technique, and award credit accordingly. Food diaries, self-monitoring, behavioral analysis, increasing activity, decreasing cue saliency, snack substitution, decreasing rate of eating, reinforcement for homework and attendence, feedback about progress, and family interventions are the stock in trade of modern nutritional counseling.

The work of the following investigators in the areas indicated was relied on as source material for this manual.

C.B. Ferster is one of the pioneers in obesity research who looked into the psychological determinants of eating behaviors and proposed the model from which ultimately this program has been derived.

R.L. Hagen has explored the role of bibliotherapy and aversive treatments in weight control programs.

H.A. Jordan has developed materials for use in behavioral weight reduction programs, along with investigating the determinants of hunger and satiety in the thin and obese populations.

L.S. Levitz has worked with weight control program development and self-help programs for the obese.

M.J. Mahoney has extensively investigated the cognitive aspects of hunger, eating, and satiety, and has systematicaly explored the basic postulates underlying the behavioral treatments of obesity.

R.W. Malott and *Behaviordelia, Inc.* provided my introduction to the behavioral techniques of contingency management, behavior chains and alternate activities, and the elements of behavioral analysis.

J.E. Mayer demonstrated much of the basic physiology of eating and the relationship between activity levels and obesity.

W.T. McReynolds has investigated the elements of behavior therapy programs for weight control and has developed stimulus control techniques to the ultimate (e.g., removing light bulbs from patients' refrigerators).

R.E. Nesbett extensively investigated the cognitive aspects of eating behaviors and the cues for hunger and satiety.

S.B. Penick demonstrated the efficacy of behavioral methods and the worth of groups for treating obesity.

L.D. Ross investigated cue saliency and developed some of the common sense "out of sight, out of mind" cue elimination techniques.

S. Schacter devised many brilliant experiments to illustrate the effects of the environment on the eating response in humans.

R.B. Stuart is the experimenter and organizer *par excellence* of the field of obesity and weight control.

A.J. Stunkard has been both an experimenter and key theoretician in weight control for the past twenty-five years.

J.P. Wollersheim was the first person to investigate the effect of a written program like *Learning to Eat* in group therapy situations.

Susan and Orland Wooley have carried out one of the most systematic series of investigations into the mechanisms of hunger, satiety, and eating behavior.

P. Watslowick, J. Haley, S. Minuchin, and *G. Bach* have been my models for family and couple interaction and intervention as described in Lesson Sixteen.

INDEX

INDEX

Related Books on Nutrition and Fitness from Bull Publishing Co.

Child of Mine: Feeding with Love and Good Sense - Expanded Edition, by Ellyn Satter, RD, ACSW $10.95

Disease Prevention/Health Promotion: The Facts, by the Office of Disease Prevention and Health Promotion, U.S. Public Health Service, U.S. Department of Health and Human Services. $24.95

Eating for Endurance, by Ellen Coleman, RD, MA, MPH, $8.95

Exercise: The Why and the How, by Paul Vodak, $11.95

How to Get Your Kid to Eat . . . But Not Too Much, by Ellyn Satter, RD, ACSW, $1[illegible]

Managing Stress Before It Manages You, by Jenny Steinmetz, PhD, et al; leader manual $3.95, participant $9.95

Maximize Your Body Potential: 16 Weeks to a Lifetime of Effective Weight Management, by Joyce D. Nash, PhD, leader manual $3.95, participant $14.95

The Nutrition Debate: Sorting Out Some Answers, by Joan Gussow, EdD and Paul R. Thomas, EdD, RD, $10.95

The Sports Medicine Fitness Course, by David C. Nieman, DHSc, MPH, $22.95

Taking Charge of Your Smoking, by Joyce D. Nash, Ph.D., leader manual $3.95, participant $14.95

Taking Charge of Your Weight and Well-Being, by Joyce D. Nash, PhD and Linda H. Ormiston, PhD, leader manual $3.95, participant $14.95

*Prices Subject to Change Without Notice

Individual orders must be prepaid. Charge by phone, or send check including $2.00 per book shipping and handling. Add 6-1/2% sales tax if California resident to:

Bull Publishing Co.
P.O. Box 208
Palo Alto, CA 94302-0208
(415) 322-2855